Wholesome
FOOD FOR
BUSY PARENTS

Wholesome
FOOD FOR
BUSY PARENTS

Cassandra Fenaughty

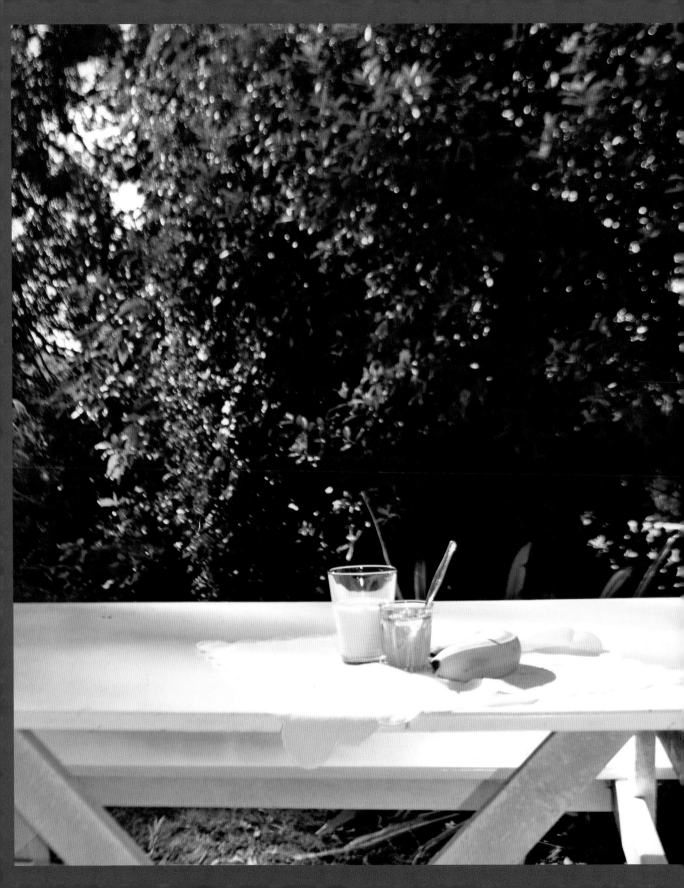

Contents

Introduction

These days being a parent is both wonderful and demanding, all at the same time! Many family units now have both parents working, children in day care, rushed mornings and evenings. Stay-at-home parents are often juggling budgets, and after a full day at home entertaining, educating and feeding children, dinner is often the last thing on their mind. So many parents tell me how tired they are, how they want to find ways to reduce their weekly grocery bill and how they know feeding their children packaged processed food isn't what they want to do, but it seems to be the only way.

Every family is different, as is every child. But through my classes I meet parents, grandparents and carers all with one thing in common – they just want what is best for their children.

Home cooking is often daunting, comments like: "I don't have the time", "I don't know how to", "Surely it's more expensive" are common, but by the end of my 90 minute class it's always a different story. *Wholesome Food for Busy Parents* shares recipes that are quick and easy, can be made in advance, and can save you money. Some recipes are new, healthier versions of everyday favorites, some are healthy cheat's versions of popular meals, and others are budget-wise recipes that use leftovers to make our lives that little bit easier.

Wholesome Food for Busy Parents provides a range of recipes that are:
- easy, with everyday and readily available, inexpensive ingredients;
- a great alternative to 'on the go' foods—with many recipes designed to be made in larger quantities to freeze and thaw as needed;
- free from refined sugar, low in salt and added fats and free from artificial colors, flavors and preservatives;
- full of goodness from wholesome fresh foods.

A last word I always leave my class parents and carers with is to just take one step at a time. If you are fortunate enough to start healthy family eating habits with your first child's first meals it will make your life easier in the long run. If your family seem to be at the other end of the spectrum, loving all of those tempting, naughty treats, just take baby steps introducing new healthy foods slowly. Write a program in your calendar of which days you are planning on eating home cooked meals and gradually increase the frequency as the months pass. It may be difficult at the start, but stay strong and like other parents who tell me how their children's behavior has changed for the better, you too will find these types of changes, while saving money and feeling better yourself.

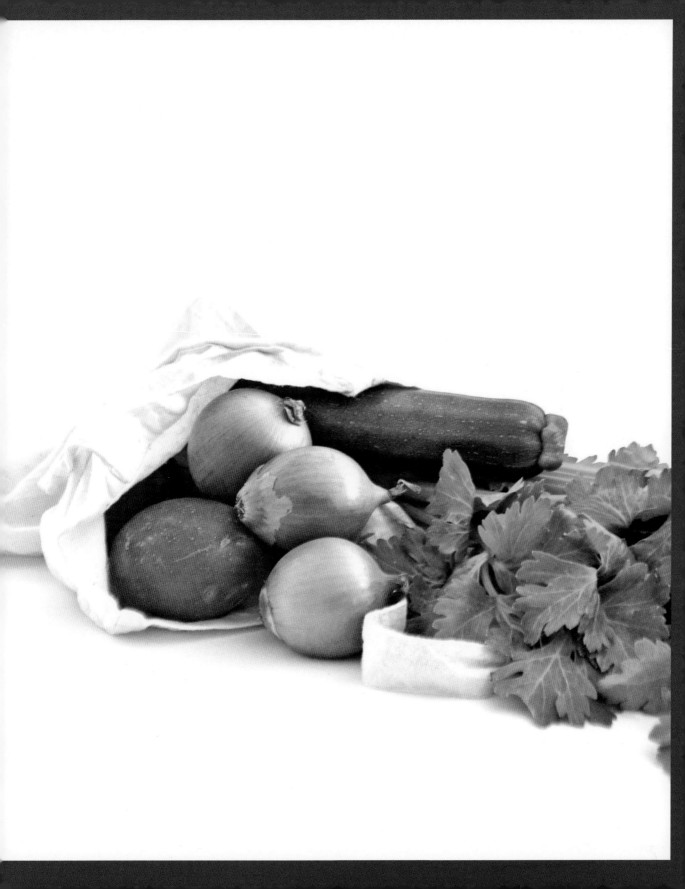

CHAPTER 1

Tips

Hints and tips are often known, sometimes forgotten but as a parent always appreciated! This chapter touches on basics such as food staples, fats, sugars and salts, storage, equipment and measurement conversions. The '2 weeks worth of snacks in 90 minutes' feature helps introduce the idea of batch cooking to home cooks.

Grocery Staples

The following ingredients aren't every ingredient listed in the book, but will form the basis of most recipes and will be enough for many of the recipes. Whilst the recipes in this book call for certain fruits and vegetables, don't be afraid to substitute with what's in season to save money and try something different – just try to keep the measures of the items the same. It's a good idea to gain familiarity with grocery items from your local supermarket that are free from preservatives, artificial colors and flavours. Organic varieties are best for dried fruits and coconut as the drying process is chemical free.

In the Pantry

Wholemeal self-raising (self-rising) flour

Cornflour (cornstarch)

Rolled oats

Quick cook oats

Baking powder

Dates

Prunes

Sultanas

Shredded coconut

Honey (low GI honey, pick your favorite type)

Cacao or cocoa powder

Passata (pureed tomatoes)

Sweet chilli sauce

Soy sauce

Pasta (wholemeal is preferred)

Long grain rice (brown is preferred)

Arborio rice

Good quality vegetable spread (yeast extract) without preservatives and added extras and low in salt

Coconut milk

Assorted dried herbs and spices

Breadcrumbs (toasted wholemeal bread blended in a food processor is preferable, if buying store bought check the ingredients for the healthiest option. Cornflake style crumbs are usually free from preservatives and additives and provide a golden crust without having to fry food in oil and butter. Homemade breadcrumbs are best stored in the freezer.)

In the Fridge

Fresh seasonal fruits

Fresh seasonal vegetables

Onions and garlic

Eggs

Milk

Greek style yogurt

Vanilla bean paste

Grated cheese (this can also be stored in the freezer)

Peanut butter (100% peanuts is preferred)

In the Freezer

Frozen corn kernels

Chopped spinach

Frozen cauliflower

Frozen berries

Mince

Chicken (free-range and organic is best if you can afford it)

Wholemeal bread (choose a brand that is free from artificial colors, flavors and preservatives)

Allergies and Substitutions

Allergies are a growing concern in our society today. Most parents with children who have allergies or intolerances are familiar with substitutions that work. Gluten-free flours and breads, milk substitutes and lactose-free cheeses and yogurts are all now readily available in the supermarket and can be used in these recipes where needed. Only a few recipes contain tree nuts and/or peanuts, feel free to substitute these at your discretion with alternative ingredients such as pan-browned rolled oats or sunflower seeds. If your child has an egg allergy, hydrated chia seeds make a great egg substitute.

Full Fat or Low Fat?

At the time of printing this book, it is not recommended to choose low fat foods or diets for infants and young children, as fat is an essential source of energy at this age and is also required for nervous system development (Kristen Beck, 2015). Reduced fat milks are not suitable for children under two years, but reduced fat varieties can be introduced to older children and adolescents (National Health and Medical Research Council, 2003). This does not mean that it's advised to serve your young children large amounts of fatty food, it simply means choose full fat dairy options and provide your child with foods containing healthy fats such as avocados, nuts and fish. It is still important to minimize saturated fats and foods with trans-fatty acids found in foods such as margarines, processed biscuits, pastries, coconut oil, meat fat and cream.

Sugar and Salt

Creating recipes for this cookbook has had its challenges. The majority of people are used to the tastes of refined sugar, highly processed grains and salty savory food. Currently there is a huge 'healthy eating' shift in our society, which is fantastic, but it also means that if we really want to be healthier, our foods will taste slightly different to what we are used to. The good news is, that once we are weaned off these highly processed foods we don't need a lot of sugar or salt to taste sweet or savory goodness. The better news is that now that we are aware and educated about the harm excess sugar and salt consumption can do to our bodies, we have the power to provide our young children with wholesome alternatives and only give them high sugar or salt foods as an occasional treat.

Whilst trialling my recipes I have come across a few comments such as "that's not sweet enough", or "I needed to add more salt". *Wholesome Food for Busy Parents* is about providing sweetness with natural and non-refined alternatives such as fruit or honey, which still contain sugars but also contain added nutrients. Salt is replaced with vegetable concentrates and cheeses, as well as herbs which add another layer of flavor. If you are used to a high sugar or salt diet, feel free to add more honey or a pinch of salt to recipes as a starting point, and then gradually reduce these elements over time. Salt and sugar are essential nutrients for our bodies, but too much can be harmful to our health.

Storage and Freezing Techniques

Once cooled, most of the dishes can be frozen quite easily. Slices and cakes can be sliced and layered in plastic or glass storage containers with layers of baking paper between them. I prefer glass containers as a healthier alternative, these are readily available now in most department and grocery stores. Ensure the glass is suitable for freezing when purchasing the containers. Purees and stews can be easily stored in washed baby jars. These are cost effective and the perfect serving size. If freezing in freezer-proof glass containers, always make sure that it is not filled to the brim to allow for any expansion in the freezer (only fill ¾ full). Simply remove from the freezer the night before and defrost in the fridge overnight for use the next day. Never put a frozen jar in a container of hot water to defrost, this will crack the glass. Always defrost slowly in the refrigerator overnight. To heat up food, leave a jar out of fridge until the chill is removed, then add warm water (not hot) to a ramekin and stir food inside the jar to warm it up. As the food warms you may add hotter water to the ramekin if necessary. Always test the temperature of food before feeding your baby.

Always ensure when cooling cooked food to freeze or use the next day as leftovers, that the food is spread thinly and evenly in a clean container, covered and placed in the fridge or freezer as soon as it cools and reaches room temperature. This is especially important when cooling and storing rice, meat and seafood. If not using the food the next day it is best to freeze. Once leftovers have been reheated or recooked in a dish, these should not be reheated or eaten again.

Equipment

Aside from general equipment such as spoons, forks, cutting boards, bowls and saucepans, the following items will be handy when home-cooking for the family:

First Foods

- Small food processor/ blender
- Storage containers for the freezer (freezer-proof glass is the healthiest option)
- Teaspoon and tea strainer for easy purees
- Glass baby food jars – large and small
- Ramekins large enough for baby food jar to fit in

Family Food

The equipment you need for first foods will continue to be of use, as well as:

- Small and if possible, a larger food processor/ blender
- Digital scales
- Measuring jug
- Combination grater including a zester grater for fine grating resulting in faster cooking
- Silicone pastry brush
- A strong fork for whisking, or a whisk, or beaters
- A correct-sized tablespoon, dessertspoon and teaspoon
- A stick blender (optional but handy)
- Large muffin tray (and a cupcake and mini-muffin tray if possible)
- Large baking tray
- Baking paper
- A lamington tin or similar 30 x 20 x 3.5 cm (13 x 10 x 2 in)
- A smaller, square baking tin 20 x 20 x 5 cm (8 x 8 x 2 in)
- A loaf tin 22 x 11 x 6 cm (9 x 4 x 3 in)

If your budget permits, other handy items in the kitchen include a rice cooker and a slow cooker, these can be purchased quite cheaply nowadays, and if treated with care will last a long time.

Two weeks of snacks in 90 minutes

Any three recipes with a stamp can be prepared and baked together in just 90 minutes. Each item can be sliced into 10–14 serves and frozen. This will provide approximately three snacks per weekday for a fortnight for one toddler or school aged child. Recipes can be doubled or tripled for more children.

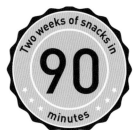

Simply wrap the snacks you need for the next day in greaseproof paper and defrost in the fridge overnight. For one child eating three snacks per day for three years, you will save a notable amount of money compared to pre-packaged toddler snacks!

By reducing takeaways for home-cooked meals your savings will double in a year if just one takeaway meal a week is replaced with a home-cooked meal.

Guide to weights and conversions

The conversions given in this book are approximate. Use the same measurement system when cooking to ensure that the proportions are consistent for each recipe.

Mass (weight)		250 g	8 oz (½ lb)
10 g	⅓ oz	280 g	9 oz
15 g	½ oz	300 g	10 oz
20 g	¾ oz	330 g	11 oz
30 g	1 oz	375 g	12 oz (¾ lb)
60 g	2 oz	410 g	13 oz
90 g	3 oz	440 g	14 oz
125 g	4 oz (¼ lb)	470 g	15 oz
150 g	5 oz (⅓ lb)	500 g (½ kg)	16 oz (1 lb)
180 g	6 oz	750 g	24 oz (1½ lb)
220 g	7 oz	1 kg	32 oz (2 lb)

Liquids (volume)		240 ml	8 fl oz
Metric	**Imperial**	300 ml	10 fl oz
30 ml	1 fl oz	375 ml	12 fl oz
60 ml	2 fl oz	400 ml	13 fl oz
90 ml	3 fl oz	440 ml	14 fl oz
125 ml	4 fl oz	500 ml	16 fl oz
150 ml	5 fl oz	750 ml	24 fl oz
180 ml	6 fl oz	1 L	32 fl oz
200 ml	7 fl oz		

Oven temperature guide				
Celsius (electric)	Celsius (fan forced)	Fahrenheit	Gas	
120°C	100°C	250°F	1	very low
150°C	130°C	300°F	2	low
160°C	140°C	325°F	3	moderately low
180°C	160°C	350°F	4	moderate
190°C	170°C	375°F	5	moderately hot
200°C	180°C	400°F	6	hot
230°C	210°C	450°F	7	very hot
250°C	230°C	500°F	9	very hot

If using a fan-forced oven, your cooking time may be a little quicker, so start checking your food a little earlier.

Cup Conversions for Metric and Imperial (Australia, New Zealand and UK Cup Measures) **Pantry**								
Ingredient	1 cup		½ cup		⅓ cup		¼ cup	
breadcrumbs*	120 g	4 oz	60 g	2 oz	40 g	1½ oz	30 g	1 oz
rolled oats	90 g	3 oz	45 g	1½ oz	30 g	1 oz	20 g	¾ oz
quick cooking oats	100 g	3⅓ oz	50 g	1¾ oz	35 g	1¼ oz	25 g	¾ oz
coconut, shredded*	60 g	2 oz	30 g	1 oz	20 g	¾ oz	15 g	½ oz
flour, plain/self-raising	150 g	4¾ oz	75 g	2½ oz	50 g	1½ oz	40 g	1½ oz
pasta spirals/penne, uncooked	90 g	3 oz	45 g	1½ oz	30 g	1 oz	20 g	¾ oz
rice, uncooked	200 g	6¾ oz	100 g	3⅓ oz	65 g	2¼ oz	50 g	1¾ oz
sultanas/dried fruit chopped*	140 g	4⅔ oz	70 g	2⅓ oz	50 g	1½ oz	35 g	1¼ oz
whole prunes or dates*	150 g	4¾ oz	75 g	2 ½ oz	50 g	1½ oz	40 g	1½ oz
mixed nuts	125 g	4 oz	60 g	2 oz	40 g	1½ oz	30 g	1 oz
red lentils dried	140 g	4⅔ oz	70 g	2⅓ oz	50 g	1½ oz	35 g	1¼ oz
rice bubbles/puffs*	30 g	1 oz	15 g	½ oz	10 g	⅓ oz	7 g	¼ oz
cornflakes*	40 g	1½ oz	20 g	¾ oz	15 g	½ oz	10 g	⅓ oz

Refrigerator and Freezer

Ingredient	1 cup		½ cup		⅓ cup		¼ cup	
cheese, shredded/grated*	120 g	4 oz	60 g	2 oz	40 g	1½ oz	30 g	1 oz
parmesan cheese, grated *	90 g	3 oz	45 g	1½ oz	30 g	1 oz	20 g	¾ oz
yogurt	260 g	8¼ oz	130 g	4 oz	90 g	3 oz	70 g	2¼ oz
1 cm (½ in) cubed vegetables*	150 g	5 oz	75 g	2½ oz	50 g	1¾ oz	40 g	1½ oz
coarsely grated fruit/vegetables*	100 g	3⅓ oz	50 g	1¾ oz	35 g	1¼ oz	25 g	¾ oz
finely grated fruit/vegetables*	150 g	5 oz	75 g	2½ oz	50 g	1¾ oz	40 g	1½ oz
pureed raw fruit/vegetables*	200 g	6¾ oz	100 g	3⅓ oz	65 g	2¼ oz	50 g	1¾ oz
steamed vegetables, chopped	140 g	4⅔ oz	70 g	2⅓ oz	50 g	1¾ oz	40 g	1½ oz
cooked pasta spirals or penne*	90 g	3 oz	45 g	1½ oz	30 g	1 oz	20 g	¾ oz
peanut butter	280 g	9 oz	140 g	4⅔ oz	95 g	3 oz	70 g	2⅓ oz
frozen corn kernels	140 g	4⅔ oz	70 g	2⅓ oz	50 g	1¾ oz	40 g	1½ oz
frozen peas*	120 g	4 oz	60 g	2 oz	40 g	1½ oz	30 g	1 oz
frozen raspberries*	90 g	3 oz	45 g	1½ oz	30 g	1 oz	20 g	¾ oz
frozen blueberries*	120 g	4 oz	60 g	2 oz	40 g	1½ oz	30 g	1 oz
frozen cauliflower florets*	120 g	4 oz	60 g	2 oz	40 g	1½ oz	30 g	1 oz

* Note: Ingredient weights may vary depending on type or size of fruit or vegetable, brand or type of dry food. Usually the differences are not large enough to affect the quality of the dish being prepared, however weight measurements are the most accurate.

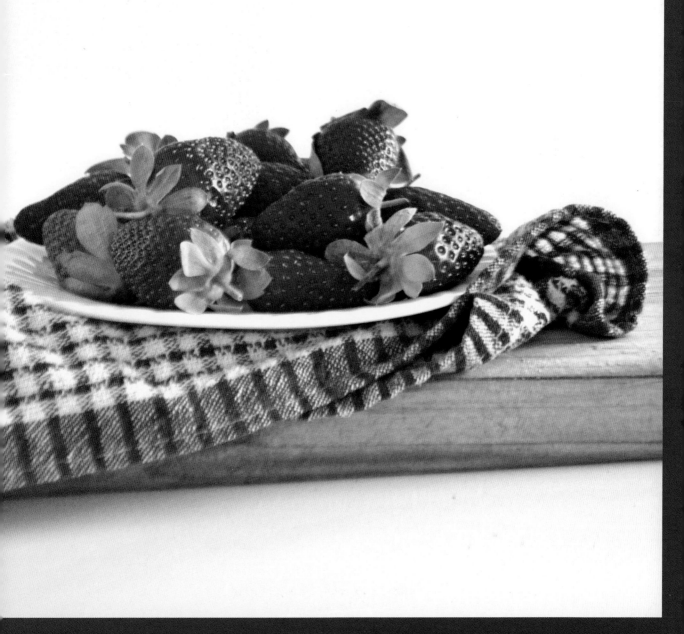

CHAPTER 2

First Foods

Starting solids with your baby, especially your first child is often exciting and fun. It is however important to speak with your midwife to ensure the timing is right, and the foods you give your baby are appropriate. Whilst there are times that packaged food is the only option, I believe that homemade is always best.

Purees

At the very beginning, I found that mixing half breast milk, half fruit or vegetables was the best way to transition my baby to solids. I always warmed the mixture to body temperature in a glass jar that was placed in a ramekin of hot water to avoid the use of plastics. As the quantity of fruit or vegetables is so small to begin with, the easiest way to puree the foods is often through a tea strainer with the back of a teaspoon.

Common favorites of the babies in our mothers group included:

- Pureed Pear: The pear can be either raw and ripe or stewed. Ensure all peel and core is removed.
- Pureed Pumpkin: Peel and remove seeds, steam until falling apart.
- Prune Juice: Pit and halve organic prunes, place in a small saucepan, cover with purified water and boil until the prunes begin to fall apart and the water is light brown. Strain and use the water with young babies, once the baby gets a bit older the prunes and water can be blended and eaten plain or with other pureed fruits or vegetables. Prunes are excellent to help constipated babies' bowels move.

These were mixed with either breast milk or formula in the beginning, then eaten plain as the babies adjusted to solids.

No Cook Purees

These purees are quick and simple for babies who are transitioning from purees mixed with breast milk or formula to straight food purees. These recipes can be made away from home if you pack a small mesh tea strainer and a metal teaspoon with the food. Quantities can be increased for older babies.

Pear and Avocado
This puree is quite runny and sweet, a great 'milk free' puree.

¼ of a ripe pear
1 tablespoon of ripe avocado flesh

1. Peel and dice pear and dice avocado.
2. Mash the pear and avocado through a mesh strainer and mix well.

Banana and Berry
The blueberry skin will remain in the strainer – discard this for babies who have just started solids. This puree is a little thicker and a good bridging consistency to lumpy foods.

¼ of a ripe small banana
4 frozen blueberries (defrosted)

1. Peel and dice the banana.
2. Mash the banana and blueberries through a mesh strainer and mix well.

Strawberry and Pear
This is a great runny and sweet puree. Always ensure strawberries are washed really well, unless organic, strawberries are usually sprayed heavily with pesticides.

1 ripe strawberry
¼ ripe pear

1. Peel and dice pear and top and dice strawberry.
2. Mash the pear and strawberry through a mesh strainer and mix well.

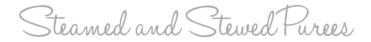

Steamed and Stewed Purees

These purees make approximately 150 ml (5 fl oz) each. Serve fresh and at room temperature or spoon into a silicone ice-cube tray or freezer-proof containers and freeze for an easy meal. A hand held mixer and a small jug can also be used for blending.

Sweet Greens
4 florets of broccoli
60 g (2 oz) frozen peas
1 ripe pear, peeled and cored

1. Steam the broccoli and peas until the broccoli is very soft and beginning to fall apart. You can also use leftover greens from dinner the night before.
2. Puree steamed vegetables and pear in a food processor until smooth.

Two Veg Favorite
2 x 1 cm (½ in) slices of a medium sweet potato
3 medium cauliflower florets (fresh or frozen)

1. Steam sweet potato and cauliflower until very soft and beginning to fall apart. You can also use leftover sweet potato with frozen cauliflower that has been defrosted.
2. Puree in a food processor until smooth.

An Apple a Day
1 large red apple peeled, cored and sliced thinly
1 carrot, grated

1. Place sliced apple and grated carrot into a small saucepan. Cover with water and bring to boil.
2. Simmer for approximately 10 minutes until apple and carrot are soft.
3. Puree in a food processor until smooth.

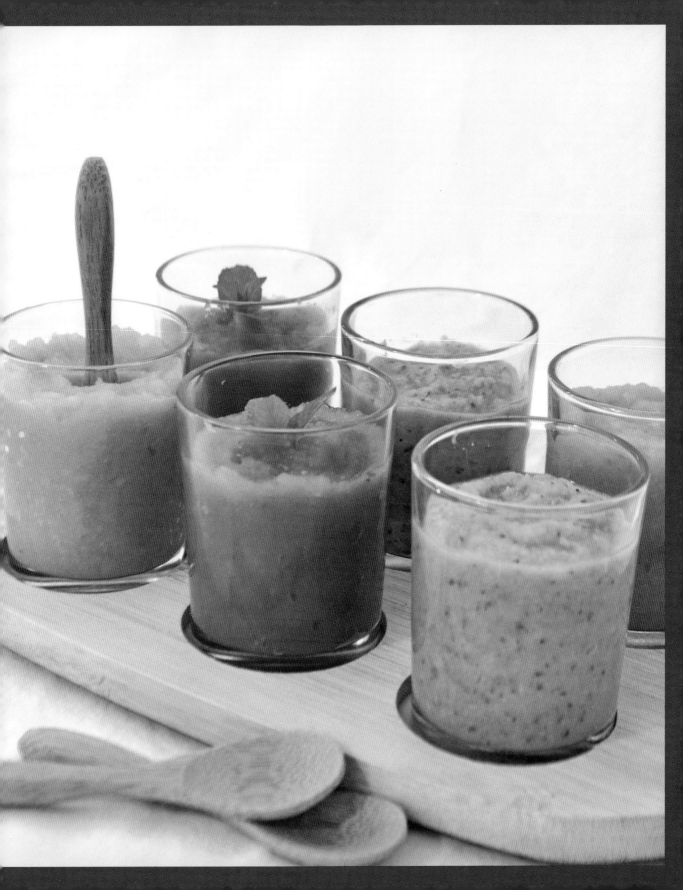

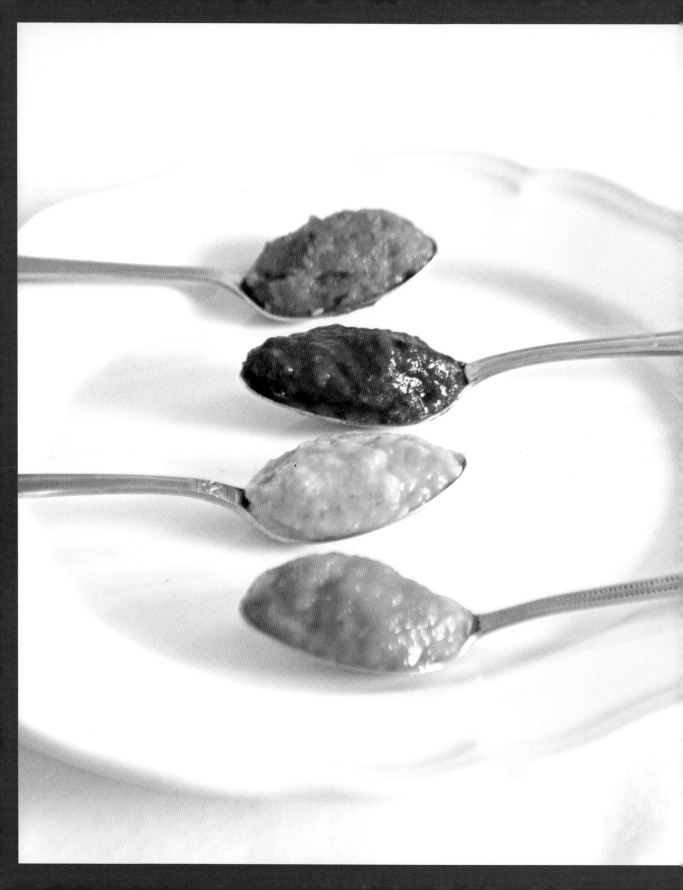

Tummy Treat

This puree is ideal for constipated babies and toddlers, always remember to offer lots of water to babies with constipation too.

4 organic pitted prunes
boiling water
4 heaped tablespoons steamed pumpkin

1. Place prunes in a small ramekin or mug and pour boiling water to cover.
2. Cool to room temperature and place in fridge overnight. This process hydrates the prunes.
3. Steam pumpkin, or use leftover pumpkin from the night before.
4. Place prunes and half of the prune infused water along with the steamed pumpkin in a food processor and puree until smooth. Add extra prune infused water for a thinner consistency.

Bananarama

3 x 1 cm (½ in) slices of sweet potato
1 small ripe banana

1. Steam sweet potato, or use leftover sweet potato from the night before.
2. Place in food processor with peeled banana and blend until smooth.

Zumpkin

This puree is a great 'all vegetable' option for first foods as it's not too thick and the pumpkin provides sweetness without the addition of fruit.

½ small zucchini (courgette)
4 heaped tablespoons steamed pumpkin

1. Steam vegetables until soft, or use leftovers from the night before.
2. Place in food processor and blend until smooth.

Green Machine

This puree is a good introduction to avocado for beginners.

½ red apple, peeled and cored, thinly sliced
½ small zucchini (courgette), thinly sliced
2 tablespoons ripe avocado

1. Place sliced apple and zucchini into a small saucepan. Cover with water and bring to boil.
2. Simmer for approximately 10 minutes until apple and zucchini are soft.
3. Allow to cool and place in food processor with avocado and blend until smooth.

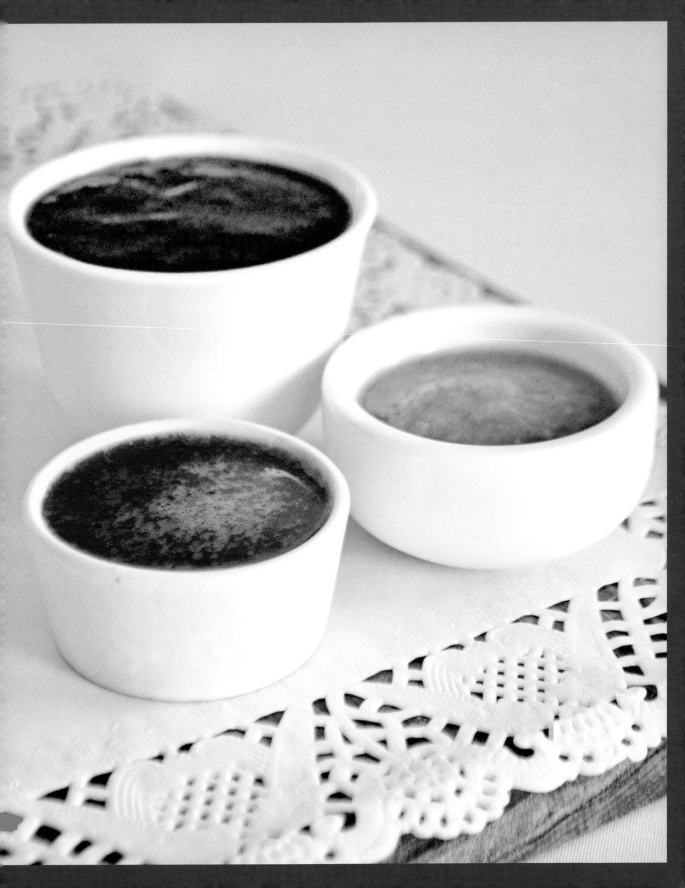

CHAPTER 3

Savory Snacks

Savory snacks are a fantastic way to incorporate a variety of vegetables, proteins and dairy into the family diet. Many parents may think their children prefer sweet snacks, however upon trialling a few different savory options they are often pleasantly surprised. The savory recipes in this chapter range from snacks to small meals and party foods.

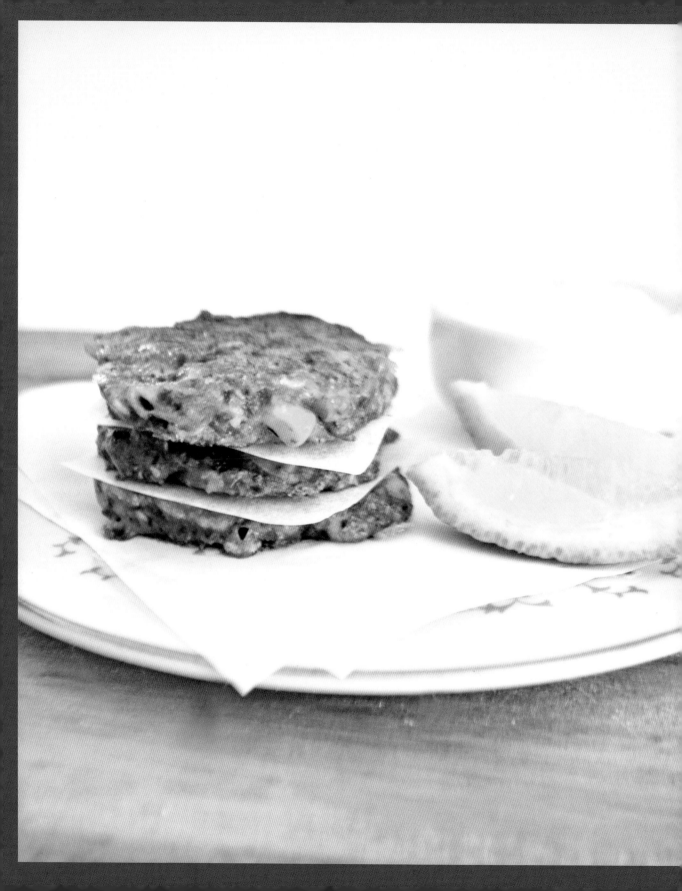

Fritters

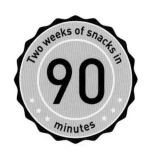

MAKES 12–15

These are great served warm or cold for snacks, or as a canapé with half a cherry tomato on top for parties. Fritters can also be frozen for a quick on-the-go or lunchbox snack.

125 g (4 oz) of chopped frozen spinach (defrosted in the fridge the night before)

1 egg

75 g (2½ oz) wholemeal self-raising flour

70 g (2⅓ oz) corn kernels, frozen or fresh

90 g (3 oz) cheese, grated

½ small onion, finely chopped

60 ml (2 fl oz) milk

Cream cheese or Greek style yogurt to serve

1. Place spinach and egg into a small blender and puree.
2. Transfer puree into a large mixing bowl and add and mix the remaining ingredients.
3. Heat a non-stick frypan on a medium heat and using a dessertspoon, spoon mixture into pan.
4. Once browned on one side, flip over and cook on other side.
5. Serve with cream cheese or Greek style yogurt.

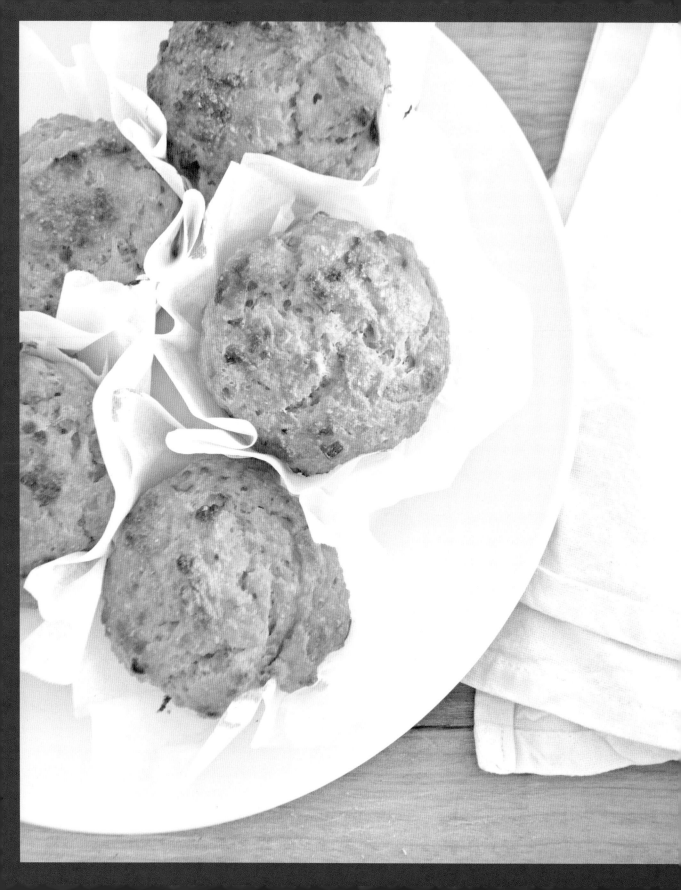

Pumpkin and Cheese Muffins

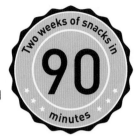

MAKES 12 MUFFINS

These muffins can be frozen for school lunchboxes or warmed up and spread with cream cheese for afternoon tea.

300g peeled and seeded pumpkin, cubed roughly

40 g (1 oz) grated cheese

45 g (1½ oz) parmesan cheese, grated

300 g (9½ oz) wholemeal self-raising flour

210 g (6¾ oz) Greek style yogurt

2 eggs

1 heaped teaspoon finely chopped onion

1 teaspoon honey

1. Preheat oven to 180°C/160°C fan forced (350°F/gas 4) and line a muffin tin with paper cases.
2. Place pumpkin into a blender and puree, if pumpkin is too dry to blend add some of the yogurt.
3. Place puree into a mixing bowl and add remaining ingredients, mix well.
4. Spoon into muffin cases and bake for 30 minutes.
5. Serve warm or cool.

Parmesan and Kale Twists

MAKES 10 TWISTS

Serve freshly baked for parties or pre-dinner snacks.

100 g (3 1/3 oz) wholemeal self-raising flour

120 g (4 oz) Greek style yogurt

4 heaped tablespoons fresh kale leaves, finely chopped

4 heaped tablespoons parmesan cheese, grated

1 egg, whisked well

Extra wholemeal flour for rolling

1. Preheat oven to 180°C/160°C fan forced (350°F/gas 4) and line a large baking tray with baking paper.
2. Mix flour and yogurt in a bowl to form a dough.
3. Turn out onto a lightly floured bench and divide into 10 portions.
4. Roll each portion out into a sausage shape approximately 20 cm (8 in) long and 1 cm (1/2 in) in diameter.
5. Place lengths of dough into pairs, sprinkling between the pairs with kale and cheese evenly.
6. Gently twist pairs of dough together, incorporating cheese and kale, gently rolling on bench after twisting to coat dough with any kale and cheese that may be left on the bench.
7. Cut each twist in half to make a total of 10 twists.
8. Place twists onto baking tray and using a pastry brush, coat both sides with egg wash.
9. Bake for 15–20 minutes or until well browned.

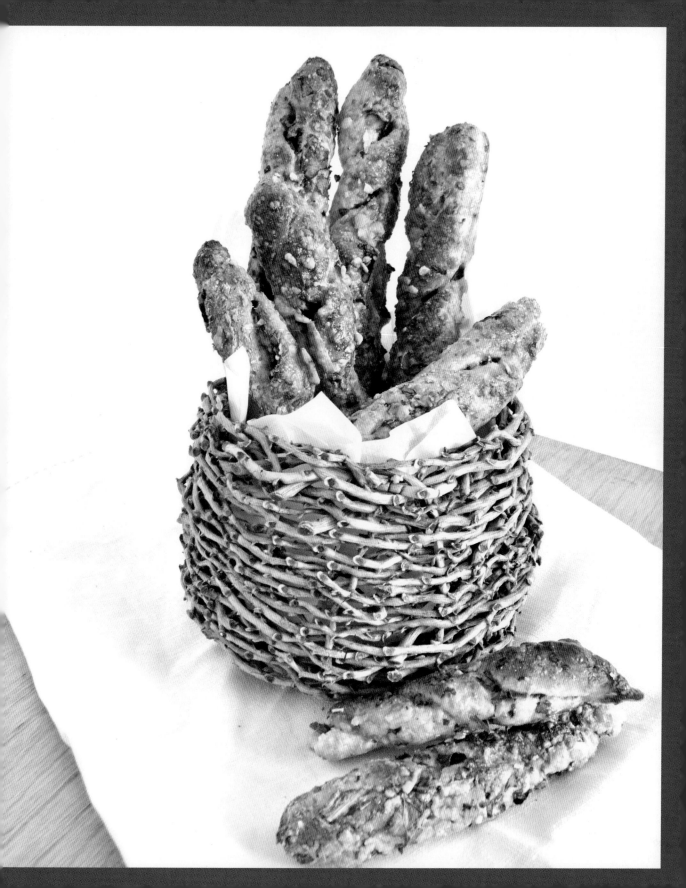

Veggie Fingers

MAKES 10-12

150 g (5 oz) finely grated vegetables
(e.g. ½ zucchini (courgette), a piece
of peeled pumpkin and ½ peeled
pear. Use vegetables that your baby
likes or needs in his/her diet. I use a
zester grater, it's easy and even hard
vegetables cook easily when grated
this fine)
1 tablespoon finely grated onion (use a
zester grater)
50 g (1½ oz) wholemeal self-raising flour
35 g (1 oz) full fat cheddar cheese,
grated
2 eggs

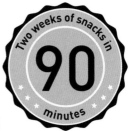

1. Preheat oven to
180°C/160°C fan forced
(350°F/gas 4) and line a
loaf tin with baking paper.
2. Mix all ingredients, pour into tin and bake
for 40–50 minutes or until firm.
3. Remove from tin and put on a rack until
cool.
4. Cut into fingers and serve. (If younger
children are finding it tricky to chew slightly
firmer foods you can slice the top and/or
sides off the loaf. I also like to place slices
in layers with baking paper between them
and freeze in a container.)

Spinach Fingers

MAKES 10-12

250 g (8 oz) packet of chopped frozen
spinach (defrosted in the fridge the
night before)
1 tablespoon finely grated onion (use a
zester grater)
50 g (1 ½ oz) wholemeal self-raising
flour
35 g (1 oz) full fat cheddar cheese,
grated
2 eggs

1. Preheat oven to
180°C/160°C fan forced
(350°F/gas 4) and line a
loaf tin with baking paper.
2. Snip the corner off the plastic spinach bag
and squeeze out excess moisture.
3. Mix all ingredients, pour into tin and bake
for 30 minutes or until firm.
4. Remove from tin and put on a rack until
cool.
5. Cut into fingers and serve.

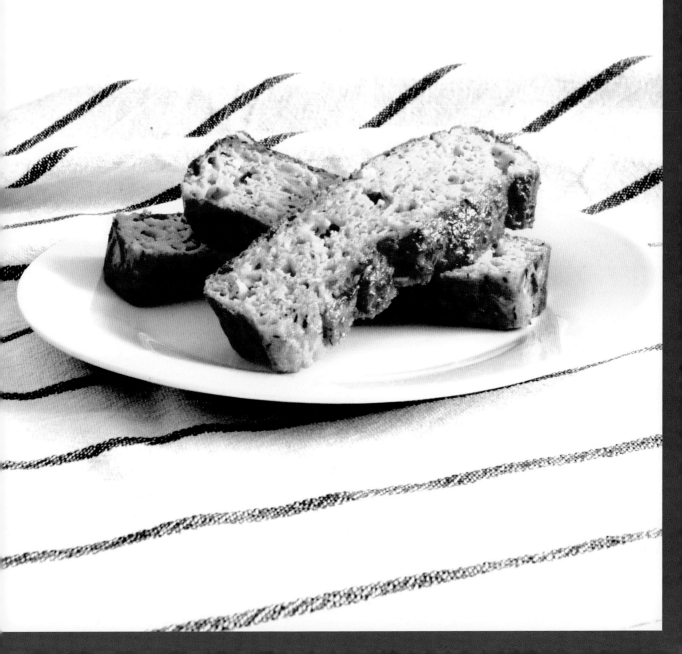

Ants on a Log

MAKES 2 SERVES

A great easy morning or afternoon tea snack. Excellent for lunchboxes too.

1–2 slices steamed zucchini (courgette) (leftovers from the night before)

1–2 steamed carrot sticks (leftovers from the night before)

1 level tablespoon steamed sweet potato or pumpkin (leftovers from the night before)

1 level tablespoon peanut butter (100% nuts preferred)

2 celery sticks

1 tablespoon organic sultanas

1. Mash or blend zucchini, carrot, sweet potato or pumpkin and peanut butter to achieve an even consistency.
2. Spread into the hollow of the celery sticks.
3. Top with sultanas and cut in half, serve.

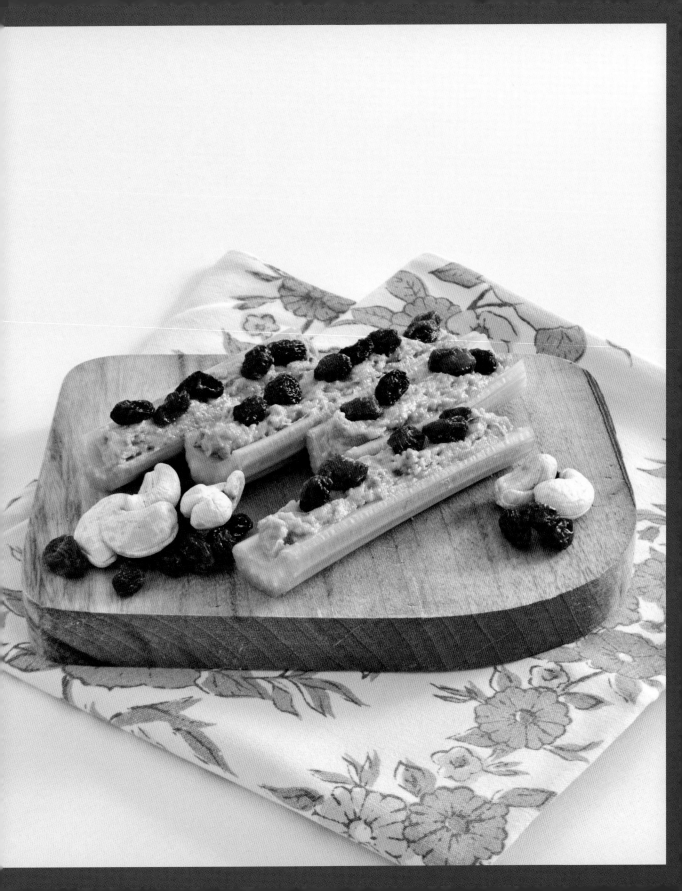

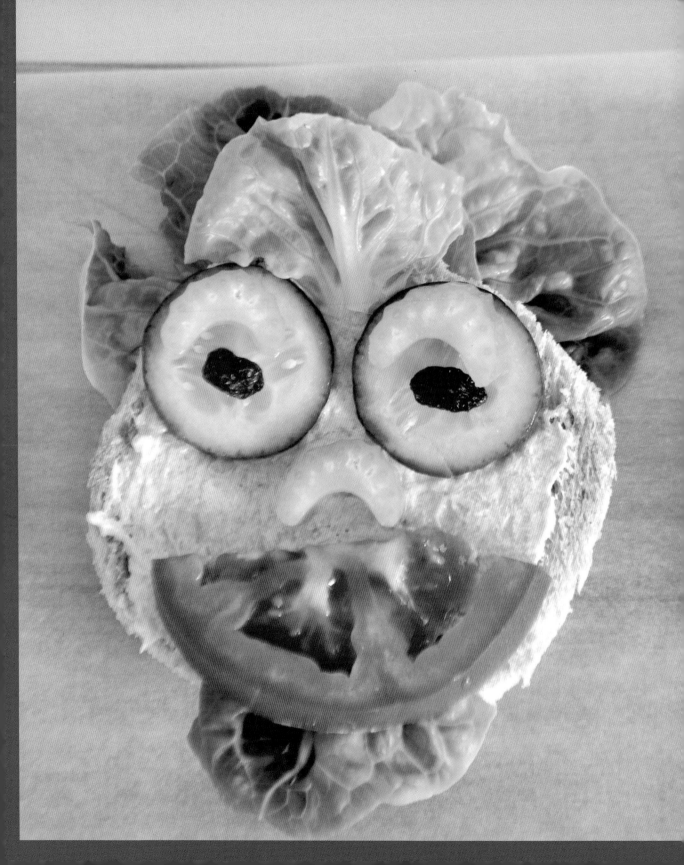

Funny Face Open Sandwiches

Yogurt mixture can be substituted with cream cheese and salad ingredients can be varied to add individuality.

2 slices of wholemeal bread
1 teaspoon leftover mashed
  pumpkin or sweet potato
2 teaspoon Greek style
  yogurt
1 slice of tomato, cut in half
6 slices of celery
4 slices of cucumber
4 organic sultanas
2 lettuce leaves

1. Cut bread slices into face-shapes or circles.
2. In a small bowl mash pumpkin or sweet potato and mix well with yogurt. Spread this mixture over the bread.
3. Place tomato on the bottom of the face for a mouth, celery for a nose and cucumber for the eyes.
4. Finish the face with celery eyebrows, sultana pupils and lettuce hair.

Pasta Salad

SERVES TWO CHILDREN FOR A QUICK AND EASY HOME OR SCHOOL LUNCH
For dinner for a family of four, simply use four times the ingredients. This is a fantastic use of leftover pasta and a nice change to sandwiches for a school lunchbox.

90 g (3 oz) cooked and cooled wholemeal pasta spirals or shells
1 heaped dessertspoon Greek style yogurt
1 tablespoon corn kernels
1 dessertspoon fresh chopped parsley and/or basil
8-10 cherry tomatoes, halved
½ avocado, diced
1 teaspoon of fresh lemon juice

1. In a medium bowl mix pasta and yogurt together until pasta well covered.
2. Add corn, herbs and tomatoes, mix through.
3. In a small bowl mix diced avocado and lemon juice, add to pasta salad and mix through carefully.

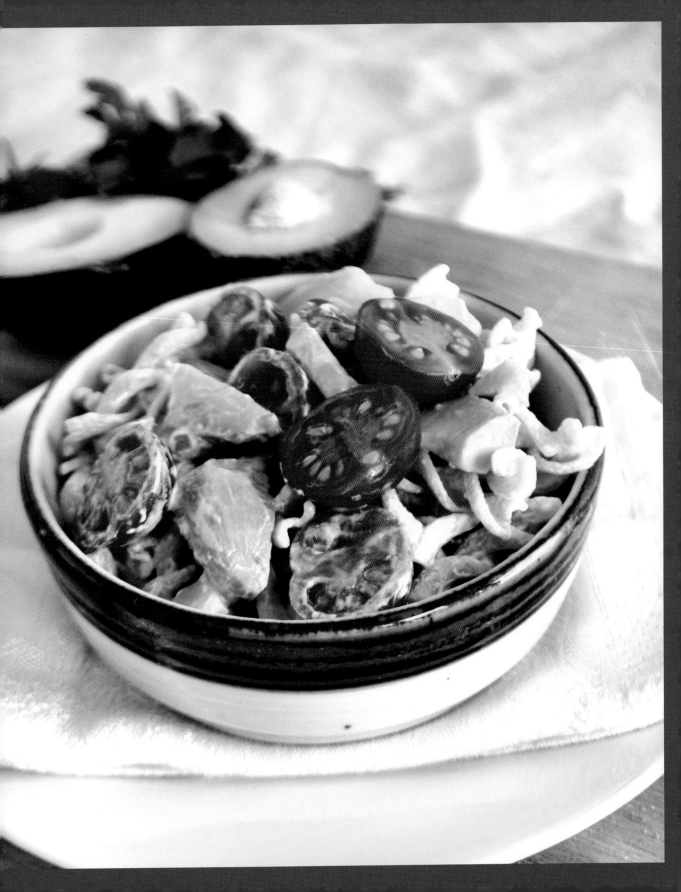

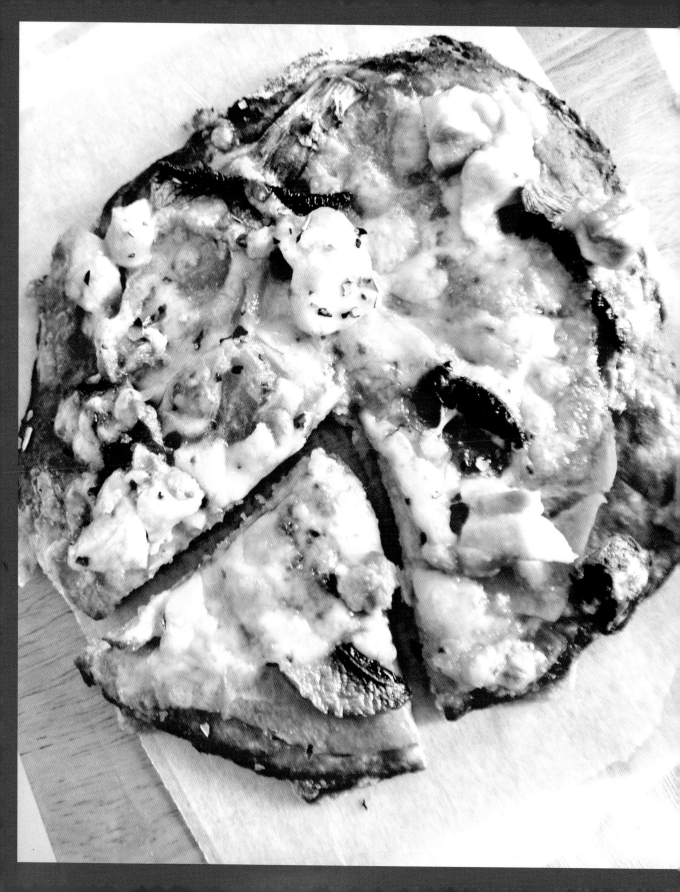

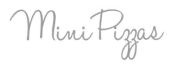

Mini Pizzas

MAKES 6

A great tasty lunch snack, or dinner with a side salad.

Toppings can be substituted with other meats and vegetables however be careful not to place too much topping on as this will affect the base cooking. Wholemeal pita pocket breads can also be used as an easy base.

Base

300 g (9 ½ oz) wholemeal self-raising flour
360 g (12 oz) Greek style yogurt

Topping

4 tablespoons passata
90 g (3 oz) pumpkin peeled and sliced very thinly (a vegetable peeler can be used if desired)
90 g (3 oz) button mushrooms sliced thinly (3-4 mushrooms)
150 g (5 oz) chicken diced very small (approx. 1 chicken thigh fillet)
80 g (2 ½ oz) cheese, grated
dried oregano or mixed herbs

1. Preheat oven to 230°C/210°C fan forced (450°F/gas 7) and line two large baking trays with baking paper.
2. Place flour in a large mixing bowl and add yogurt. Mix well.
3. Flour a clean work surface and turn out the dough then knead for a couple of minutes until smooth.
4. Divide dough into six portions, roll each portion into a bowl and roll out into a thin mini pizza base (approx. 10–12 cm (4–5 in) diameter) with a floured rolling pin or a floured tall plastic tumbler.
5. Place the bases on the baking trays and spread with passata.
6. Top with pumpkin, mushrooms, chicken, cheese and a light sprinkling of herbs.
7. Place into oven and bake for 20–25 minutes, or once cheese is golden and pumpkin slices are soft.
8. Serve warm or cold in lunchboxes.

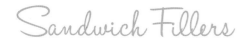

Sandwich Fillers

Once your child is ready to eat little sandwiches it is a lot easier to prepare snacks and 'on the go' lunches for them. I prefer a good quality wholemeal bread and it's easier for little ones to handle the bread with crusts cut off in the beginning. I don't believe there is a need for butter, if you feel that the bread is too dry, avocado, cream cheese or Greek style yogurt are great substitutes. Steamed and roasted vegetables will become your best friend, make extra with your evening meal and freeze in small jars to use as sandwich fillers. Below is a list of fillers that are easy and nutritious.

Cream Cheese and Jam
Homemade jam is so easy, a small ramekin can last for a few days. Defrost 2 tablespoons of frozen raspberries and mash with one ripe, peeled pear. Spread this over one slice of bread and spread cream cheese on the other. Place both slices together and cut into fingers or squares.

If you are worried about some of the ingredients in store bought cream cheese, it's quite easy to make your own. Using full fat natural or Greek style yogurt (homemade or store bought) spoon yogurt into a piece of clean muslin cloth, tie the top and hang in a large jug in the fridge overnight. The whey will drain through the cloth and leave you with firm cream cheese. Unwrap and store in an airtight container in the fridge, use within a couple of days. When hanging ensure there is sufficient room in the bottom of the jug for the whey to drain, I use a chopstick lying across the top of the jug to hang the cloth from, line it up with the spout of the jug and tie to the handle to secure it.

Pumpkin and Colby Cheese
Simply mash leftover steamed pumpkin and spread on bread, top with slices of colby cheese (or similar).

Chicken, Mango and Avocado
Blend or mash cooked chicken with fresh mango. Spread this over one slice of bread and spread avocado on the other. Place both slices together and cut as desired.

Sweet Potato, Cream Cheese and Tomato
Mash together leftover sweet potato, finely chopped tomato and a dollop of cream cheese to achieve a moist consistency. Spread on bread and serve as either an open or closed sandwich.

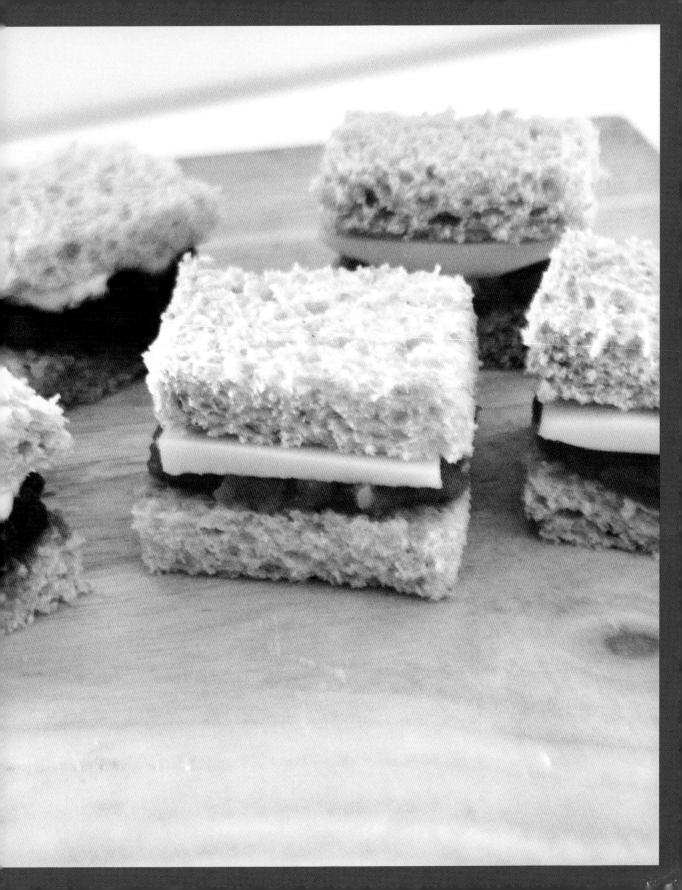

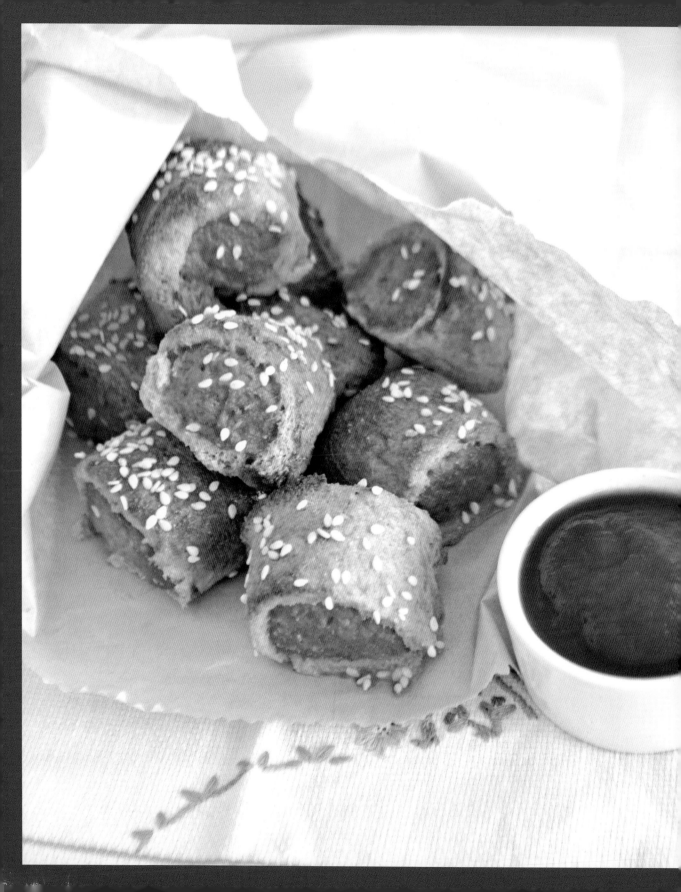

Sneaky Sausage Rolls

MAKES 24–28 MINI SAUSAGE ROLLS

A perfect party food or fun snack with friends, serve warm.

Filling

1 small carrot
40–50 g (1 ½ oz) pumpkin
½ onion
½ clove garlic
1 level teaspoon veggie
   spread (yeast extract) or
   similar
2 slices of wholemeal bread
250 g (8 oz) lean beef mince
1 egg

Wrapping

6-7 slices wholemeal bread
125 ml (4 fl oz) milk
1 egg
Sesame seeds

1. Preheat oven to 180°C/160°C fan forced (350°F/gas 4) and line a large baking tray with baking paper.
2. Place carrot, pumpkin, onion, garlic and veggie spread (yeast extract) into a food processor and puree. Add bread, mince and egg and blend until well combined. Set aside.
3. Lay bread slices out on a clean work surface and using a rolling pin roll out the bread firmly. Cut off crusts.
4. Pour milk in a shallow bowl and soak rolled out bread slices on each side.
5. Lay soaked bread on clean board and spoon a thin sausage shaped length of mince mixture down the center of each slice. Put enough mince mixture in so that when the bread wraps over the mince the edges join and do not overlap. Be careful not to overfill.
6. Place long sausage rolls join-side down on baking tray and cut into 4 mini sausage rolls each.
7. Whisk egg and brush sausage rolls with a generous egg wash. Follow with a light sprinkling of sesame seeds.
8. Bake in oven for 20–30 minutes.

Mini Hot Dogs

SERVES TWO ADULTS AND TWO YOUNG CHILDREN FOR A FUN LUNCH OR EASY DINNER
Capsicum (peppers) can be used instead of mushrooms if preferred.

6 small wholemeal bread rolls

6 small organic/ preservative free sausages (or tofu sausages)

Topping

1 small onion, diced

2 ripe tomatoes, diced

8 button mushrooms, sliced

3 heaped tablespoons pumpkin, grated

1 large avocado

80 g (2 ½ oz) cheese, grated

1. Cut half of the way through each bread roll. Lay out the rolls on grill tray and set aside.
2. In a large frypan sauté the onion in a little olive oil until transparent.
3. Turn heat down to medium and add tomatoes, mushrooms and grated pumpkin. Stir through and cover, stirring occasionally until tomatoes and pumpkin are soft and onions begin to caramelize. Set mixture aside.
4. Fry or grill sausages until cooked through.
5. Assemble hot dogs by spreading avocado on rolls, placing sausages, spooning tomato and onion mixture over sausages and topping with grated cheese.
6. Grill or bake in a hot oven until cheese is melted.

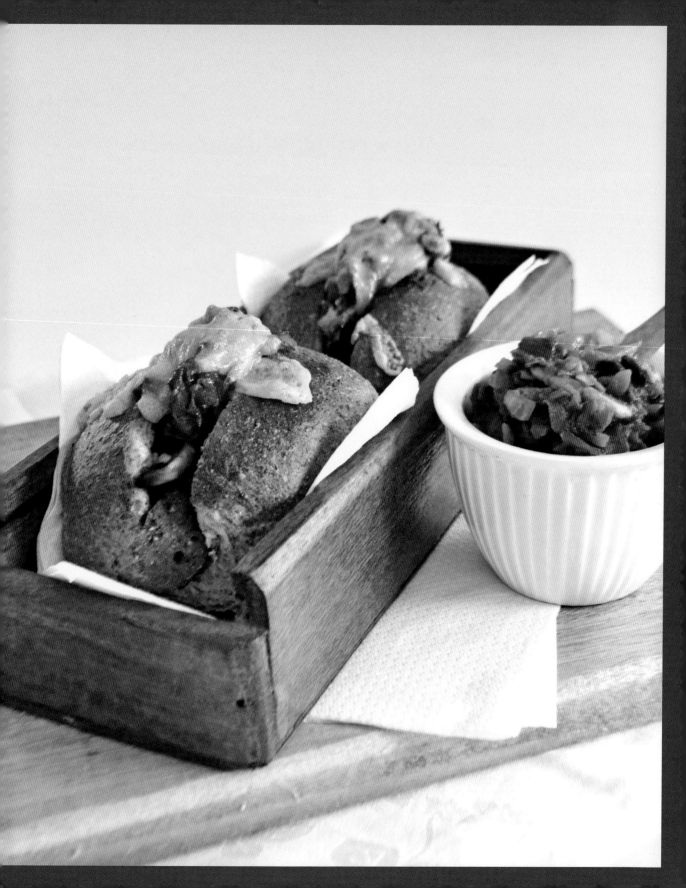

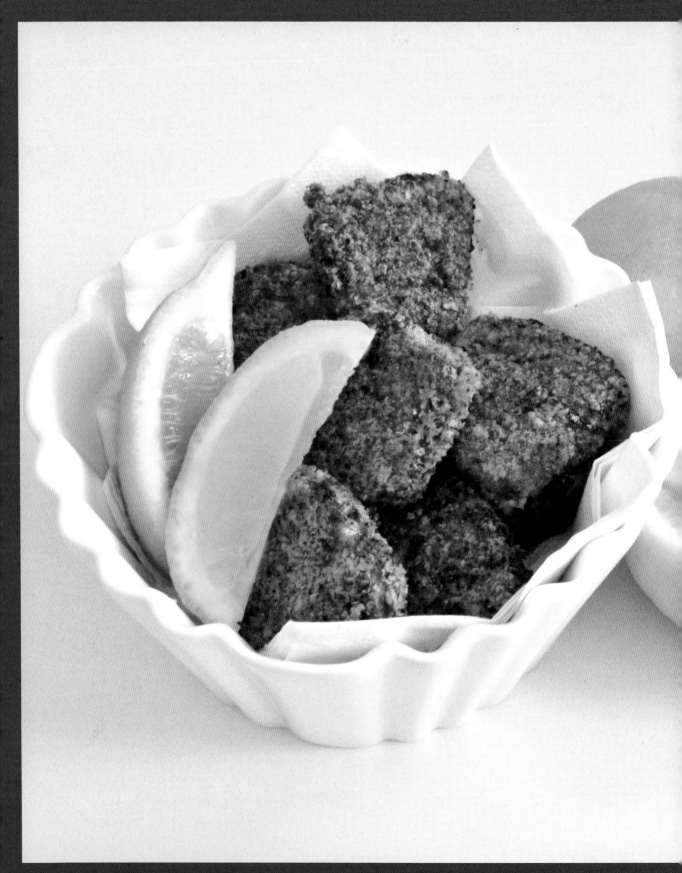

Chicken Nuggets

The quantity can be increased and frozen in an airtight container after crumbing. The nuggets can also be baked on a tray with baking paper in a moderate oven until firm and cooked through.

For variety finely grated parmesan cheese can be added to the breadcrumbs, or pureed vegetables can be added to the egg mixture.

2 large eggs, whisked
   lightly
150–180 g (4¼ oz)
   breadcrumbs
200–250g (8 oz) free range
   chicken stir-fry strips
   (tenderloins can be used
   too)

1. Lay out a bowl containing the whisked eggs, a plate with the breadcrumbs spread evenly and another plate with paper towel on it.
2. Using kitchen scissors, cut fresh chicken stir-fry strips in half to form nugget-like shapes.
3. Dip each piece of chicken in the egg, then place and turn in the crumbs to ensure they are covered. Repeat the process to double-crumb each nugget.
4. Once all nuggets are double-crumbed, place on the paper towel, cover plate in cling film and refrigerate until cooking time.
5. Pre-heat a non-stick frypan and fry nuggets on a medium heat on both sides until they begin to brown. (It is always a good idea to cut one open to ensure the chicken is cooked through before serving.)
6. Serve with lemon wedges as a snack or with chunky chips and salad as a meal.

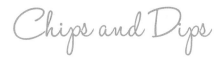
Chips and Dips

SERVES 4
Serve both dips cold with chips and vegetable sticks.

Moroccan Dip
3 tablespoons cooked (leftover) pumpkin and/or sweet potato
130g (4 oz) Greek style yogurt
large pinch ground cumin seeds
large pinch ground coriander seeds
⅓ teaspoon honey

1. Mash and mix through all ingredients until smooth.

Greek Dip
1 small zucchini (courgette), grated finely and then chopped roughly
130 g (4 oz) Greek style yogurt
¼ teaspoon raw garlic, grated finely
2 teaspoons lemon juice

1. Mix through until well combined.

Chips
Wholemeal pita or Lebanese breads

1. Cut two wholemeal pita or Lebanese breads into fingers or triangles with kitchen scissors.
2. Lay flat in non-stick frypan on medium heat until crunchy on one side. Turnover and repeat. These can also be cooked in a moderate oven until crunchy.

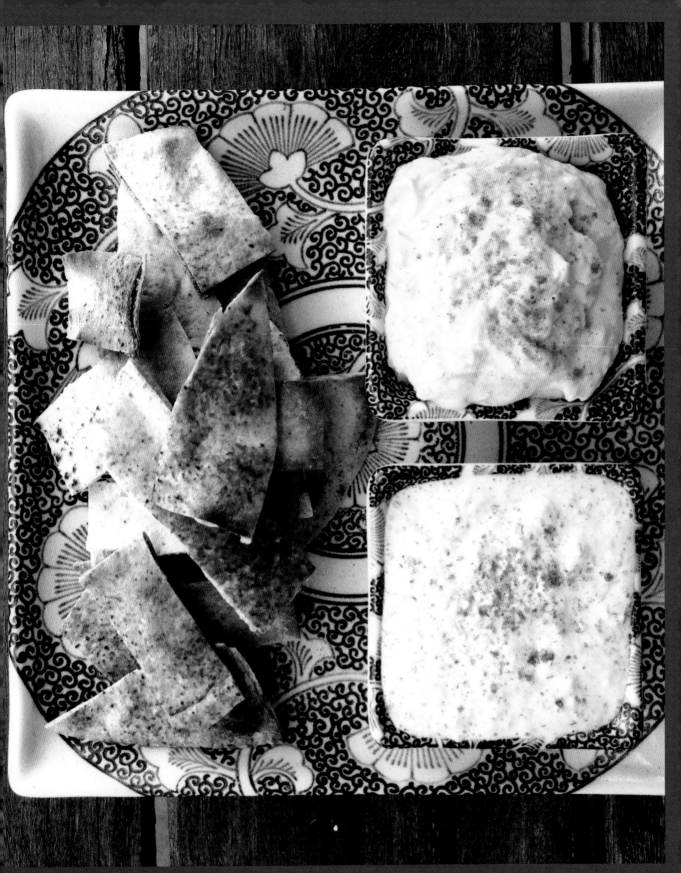

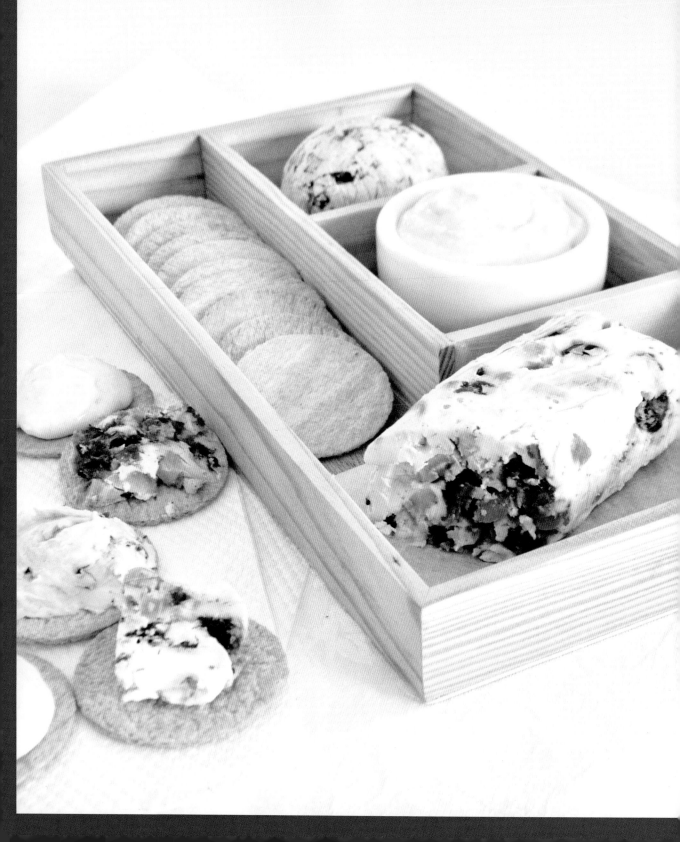

Cream Cheese Trio

This cheese trio is ideal for special occasions when entertaining other children and adults. Serve with 100% brown rice crackers, carrot and celery sticks. This snack does not contain any gluten and is also free from refined sugars and added fats, however as cream cheese contains a large percentage of natural dairy fat, small serving portions are recommended.

Cheese and Chives

⅓ of a 250 g (8 oz) tub of cream cheese (check ingredients to avoid preservatives and additives)

1 heaped tablespoon chopped chives

Once cheese is at room temperature mix thoroughly in a small bowl. Line a small ramekin with cling film and press the mixture into it. Refrigerate and turn out, removing cling film once firm.

Sweetcorn Spread

3 heaped tablespoons corn kernels

1 tablespoons water

1 level teaspoon honey

⅓ of a 250 g (8 oz) tub cream cheese (check ingredients to avoid preservatives and additives)

Place corn kernels, water and honey in a small food processor and blend until smooth. Add room-temperature cream cheese and blend until well combined. Refrigerate and serve in a dipping bowl.

Date and Nut Cheese

⅓ of a 250g (8oz) tub cream cheese (check ingredients to avoid preservatives and additives)

1 tablespoon water

1 level teaspoon honey

1 heaped tablespoon mixed nuts, chopped roughly (cashews, walnuts and macadamias are great)

3 pitted dates, chopped finely

Once cheese is at room temperature mix thoroughly with water in a small bowl. Add honey, nuts and dates and mix well. Turn out onto a sheet of cling film and roll into a sausage shape, pressing down sides to form a small rectangular loaf shape. Refrigerate and turn out, removing cling film once firm.

Parmesan Popcorn

SERVES TWO AS A TASTY SAVORY TREAT

1 tablespoon of olive oil
(optional)
2 heaped tablespoons of
popcorn kernels
2 tablespoons parmesan
cheese, grated
1/8 teaspoon garlic powder
Olive oil spray

1. Pop the corn kernels in electric popcorn maker or in saucepan by heating oil in a large saucepan, test if the oil is hot enough by dropping a single kernel into the pan, once it starts moving around the oil is hot enough to put all kernels into the pan.
2. Cover immediately with the lid and wait for the corn to pop, once popping has slowed down remove from heat and wait 30 seconds prior to opening lid.
3. While the corn kernels are popping mix parmesan cheese and garlic powder in a small bowl.
4. Lightly spray popcorn with olive oil spray and sprinkle cheese mixture on top, mixing through well.

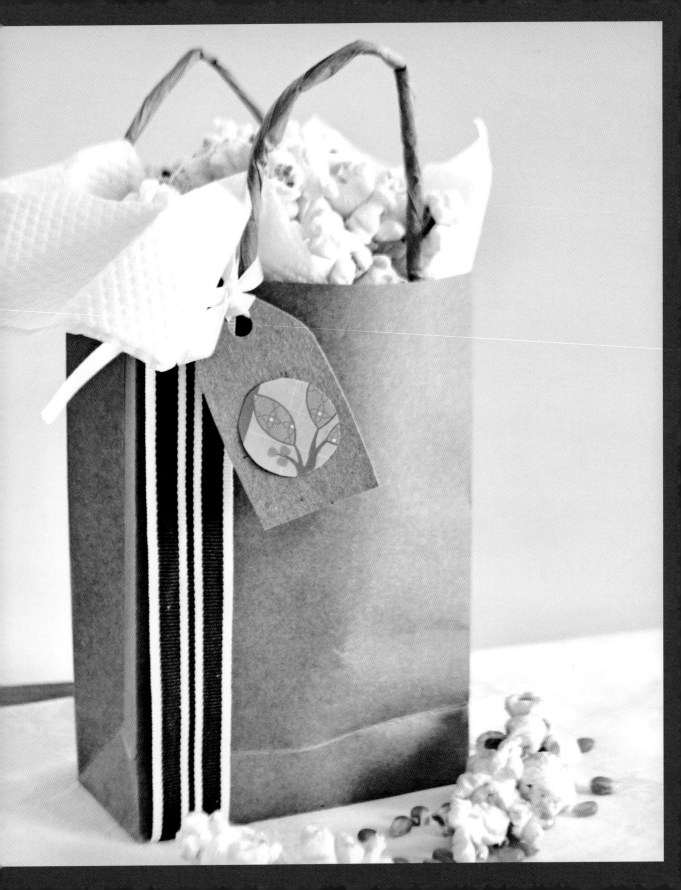

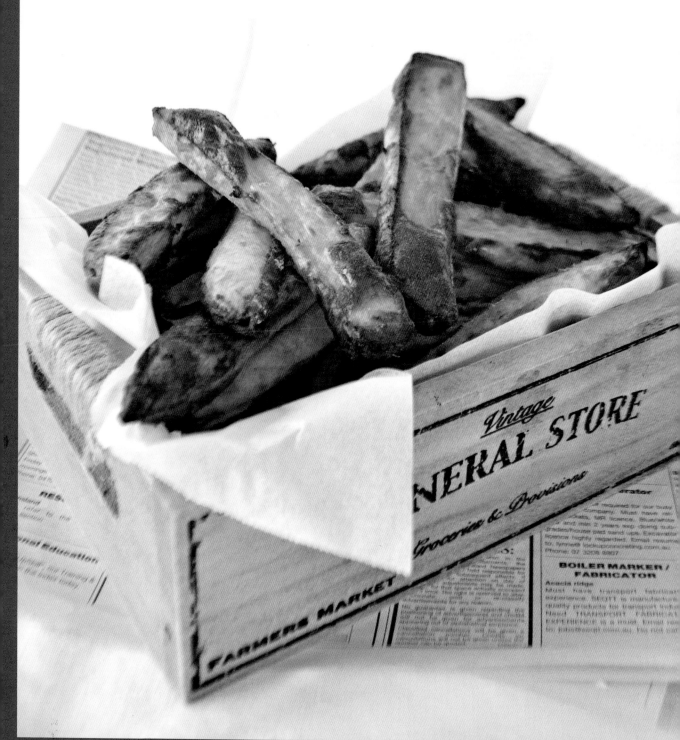

Chunky Chips

Serve these hot as a snack or side dish to an evening meal.

3 large washed potatoes
2 egg whites
1 teaspoon ground cumin
  seeds
¼ teaspoon mustard
  powder
1 teaspoon garlic powder
1 teaspoon honey

1. Preheat oven to 200°C/180°C fan forced (400°F/gas 6) and line 2 large baking trays with baking paper.
2. Leaving peel on potatoes, cut into chunky chips approximately 1–2 cm thick (½–¾ in).
3. Lay chips on a clean tea towel and pat dry.
4. While potatoes are drying, whisk egg whites, spices and honey until light but still runny.
5. Dip potatoes into egg mixture and lay onto baking trays.
6. Bake for approximately 30 minutes, or until golden brown and crunchy. Check chips after about 15 minutes to see if they need turning or rearranging in oven to cook evenly.

For extra flavour seasoning mix can be sprinkled on the chips once laid on baking tray, before putting in the oven.

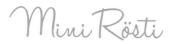

Mini Rösti

MAKES APPROXIMATELY 20 SMALL RÖSTI

These are a great snack or side to a Sunday breakfast or BBQ and salad dinner.

½ onion, diced finely

2 medium sized potatoes, grated coarsely with skin left on

1 egg

4 tablespoons wholemeal flour

2 tablespoons parmesan cheese, finely grated

1 tablespoon chopped chives

1. Mix all ingredients thoroughly in a mixing bowl.
2. Pre-heat a non-stick frypan on a medium heat. Using a dessertspoon, spoon potato mixture into frypan, flattening each rösti down to ensure even cooking.
3. Once golden brown, flip each rösti over, and turn down heat to low and cook the other side slowly to ensure potato and onion is cooked thoroughly.

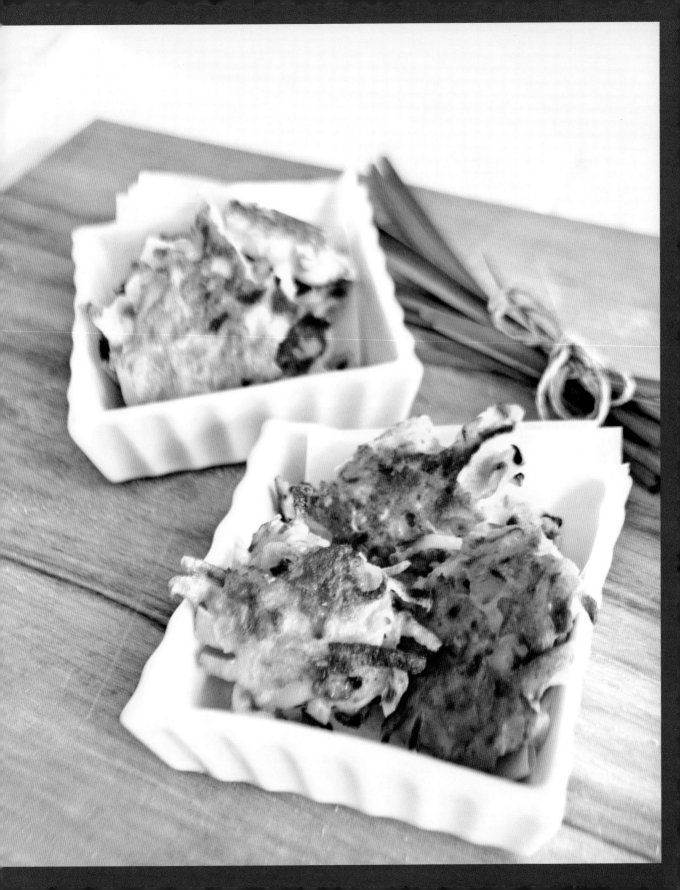

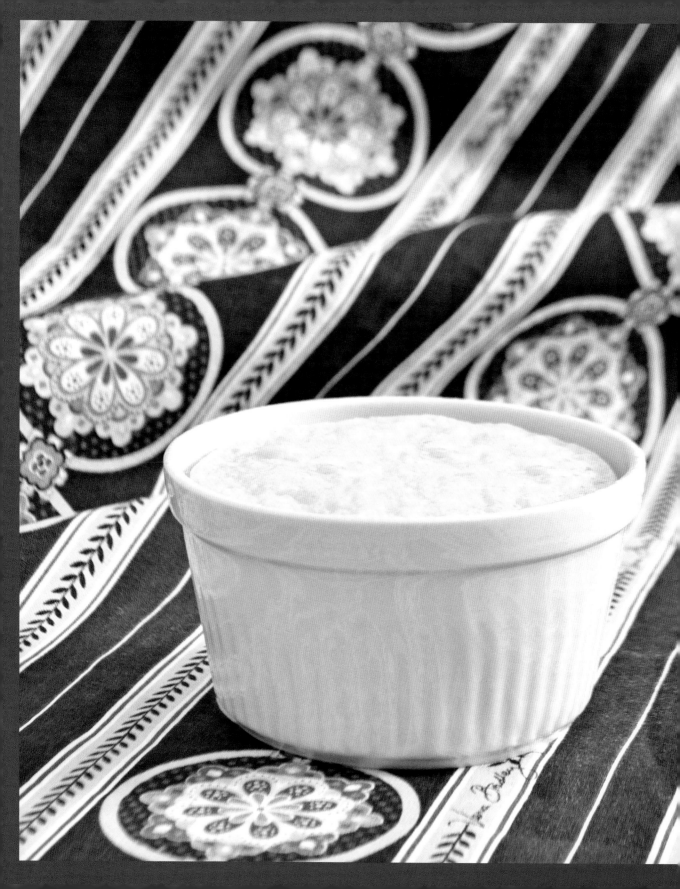

Steamed Eggie

MAKES 1

Add two tablespoons of sautéed tomato and zucchini (courgette) to mixture for variety. This dish can be eaten warm or cold the next day if stored in the fridge overnight.

1 egg

60 ml (2 fl oz) full cream milk

1 tablespoon cheese, grated

1. Lightly grease a ramekin with butter or oil.
2. Whisk egg well, then add milk and cheese and whisk together.
3. Place ramekin in empty saucepan.
4. Carefully add water to saucepan around ramekin to come up ¾ of the way up the dish.
5. Place lid on, bring to a slow boil.
6. Simmer until mixture is firm.

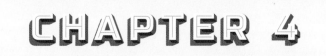

CHAPTER 4

Easy Meals

Two comments I frequently hear from parents are that they need more ideas for their children's lunchboxes, and that by the end of the day they often lack the energy to even think about what they will prepare for dinner. The Easy Meals chapter of this book is designed to free up time in our busy lives so we can spend it with our family, appreciate the food we have available to us and enjoy each other's company.

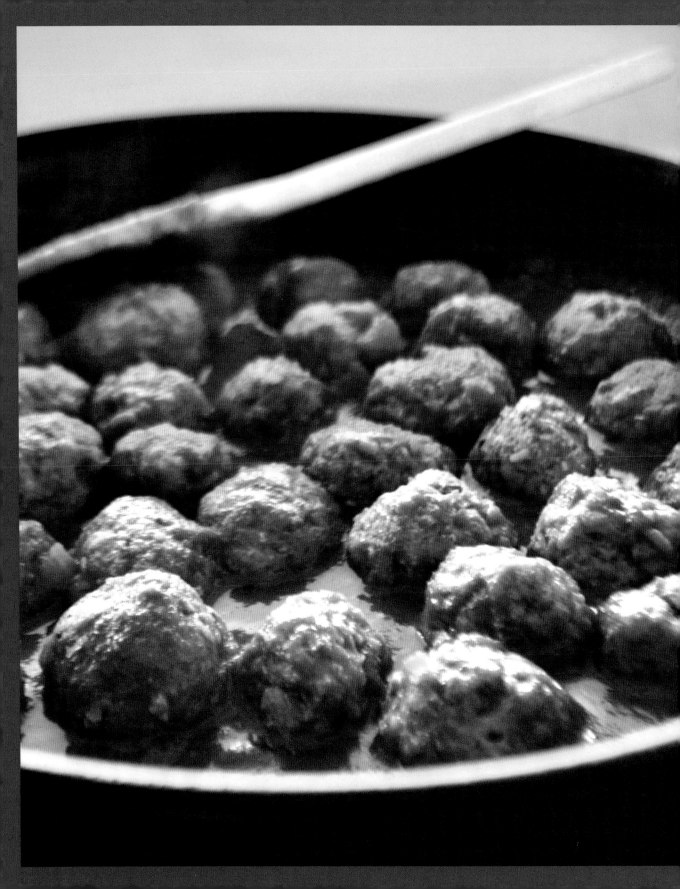

Mini Meatballs

THIS BATCH MAKES 30–40 MEATBALLS, ENOUGH FOR A FAMILY MEAL WITH LEFTOVERS FOR FREEZING
Serve with pasta, rice or mashed potato and steamed greens or salad.

Sauce

1 clove of garlic, crushed
½ onion, finely chopped
Pinch dried oregano
375 ml (12 fl oz) passata
   (tomato puree)
375 ml (12 fl oz) water

Meatballs

2 tablespoons finely
   chopped onion
400 g (13 oz) lamb mince
2 tablespoons celery leaves,
   chopped finely
40 g (1 oz) grated cheese
1 large egg whisked lightly
180–240 g (6–7 ½ oz)
   breadcrumbs

Sauce

1. In a large frypan sauté the garlic and onion in a little vegetable or olive oil.
2. Add oregano, passata and water, mix through. Bring to boil and then turn stove down to simmer. Cover pan.

Meatballs

1. In a large mixing bowl combine all meatball ingredients mixing with a wooden spoon, or hands until thoroughly mixed.
2. Roll into balls approximately 3 cm (1.2 in) in diameter and set aside on a plate.
3. Once all meatballs are rolled gently place them into the simmering sauce.
4. Replace lid and simmer for approximately 15 minutes or until cooked through.

Very Hidden Vegetable Pasta Sauce

Serve with your favorite pasta and garden salad.

280 g (9 oz) leftover
steamed vegetables
(e.g. sweet potato,
pumpkin, beans, zucchini
(courgette), carrots etc)
$\frac{1}{2}$ small onion finely diced
1 clove of garlic, minced or
finely chopped
375 ml (12 fl oz) passata
125 ml (4 fl oz) water
Pinch dried oregano or
mixed herbs

1. Puree steamed vegetables and $\frac{1}{3}$ of the passata in a food processor or blender, set aside.
2. Lightly sauté onion and garlic in a medium saucepan or frypan with a very small amount of olive or ricebran oil.
3. Add pureed vegetables and stir through over heat.
4. Add balance of passata and water and herbs, bring to boil then turn down heat to simmer for approximately 30 minutes.

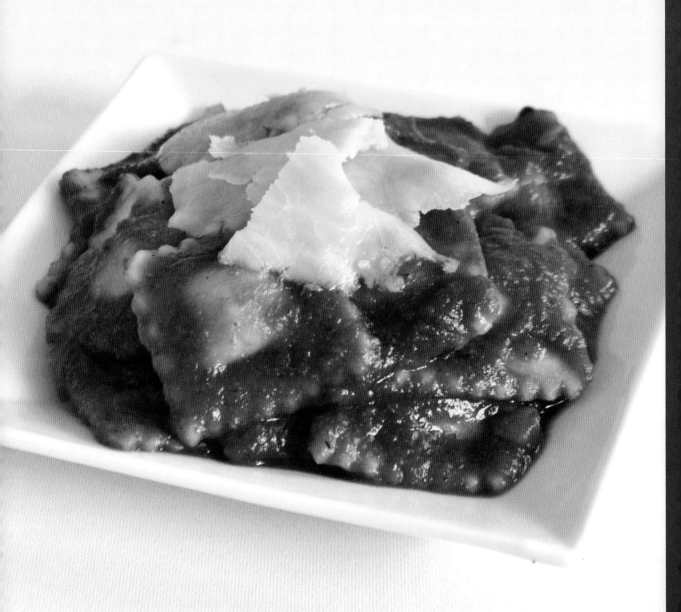

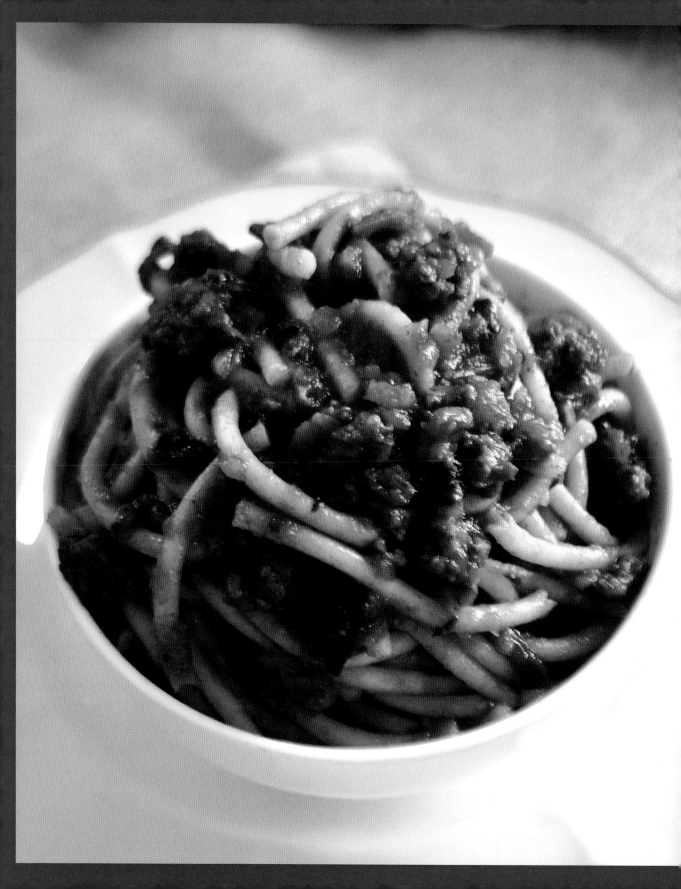

Batches O'Bolognaise

THIS RECIPE MAKES 2–3 MEALS FOR TWO ADULTS AND TWO CHILDREN
Simply freeze the remaining bolognaise in containers for quick and easy future meals.

500 g (17 ½ oz) beef mince
(or half beef, half pork)

2 onions, diced

2 cloves of garlic, minced or
finely chopped

2 large carrots, grated
finely (use a zester grater)

300 g (10½ oz) pumpkin,
grated finely (use a zester
grater)

250 g frozen chopped
spinach (frozen or
defrosted is fine)

2 heaped teaspoons
vegetable spread (yeast
extract) or similar

1 dessertspoon dried
oregano (or mixed herbs)

40 g (1⅓ oz) red lentils

500 ml (16 fl oz) passata

500 ml (16 fl oz) water

1. Brown mince and add onion in a large non-stick frypan
   or large non-stick saucepan.
2. Add garlic, carrots and pumpkin, fry turning frequently
   until vegetables begin to soften.
3. Add balance of ingredients, bring to boil then turn down
   heat, cover and simmer for at least 30 minutes.
4. Stir and simmer for another 30–60 minutes, until sauce
   has reduced and consistency is thick and rich.
5. The longer this sauce is cooked, the more flavorsome
   it will become, if necessary add a little more water if
   simmering for a longer period. This can also be made in
   a slow or multi-cooker.
6. Serve with your favorite pasta and salad.

Chicken Parmigiana

SERVES TWO ADULTS AND TWO CHILDREN

1 large egg whisked lightly
90 g (3 oz) breadcrumbs
1 large chicken breast
  200–250 g (8 oz) (thigh
  fillets can be used also)
90 ml (3 fl oz) passata
75 g (2¼ oz) grated cheese

1. Lay out a bowl containing the whisked egg, one plate with breadcrumbs spread evenly over it and another plate with paper towel on it.
2. Using kitchen scissors, cut the fresh chicken breast lengthways to create 3–4 thin fillets. Alternatively wrap the chicken in cling film and use a meat cleaver to flatten the fillet to about ½ cm (¼ in). Cut chicken fillet into 2 large and 2 small fillets.
3. Dip each piece of chicken in the egg, then place and turn in the crumbs to ensure they are covered.
4. Pre-heat a non-stick frypan and fry chicken on a medium heat on both sides until they begin to brown.
5. Once all the fillets are cooked, place in a baking dish or on a baking tray and pour passata over the chicken evenly, followed by the grated cheese.
6. Place under the grill or at the top of hot oven until the cheese is melted and golden.

Serve with a garden salad and potato or chunky chips (see page 61).

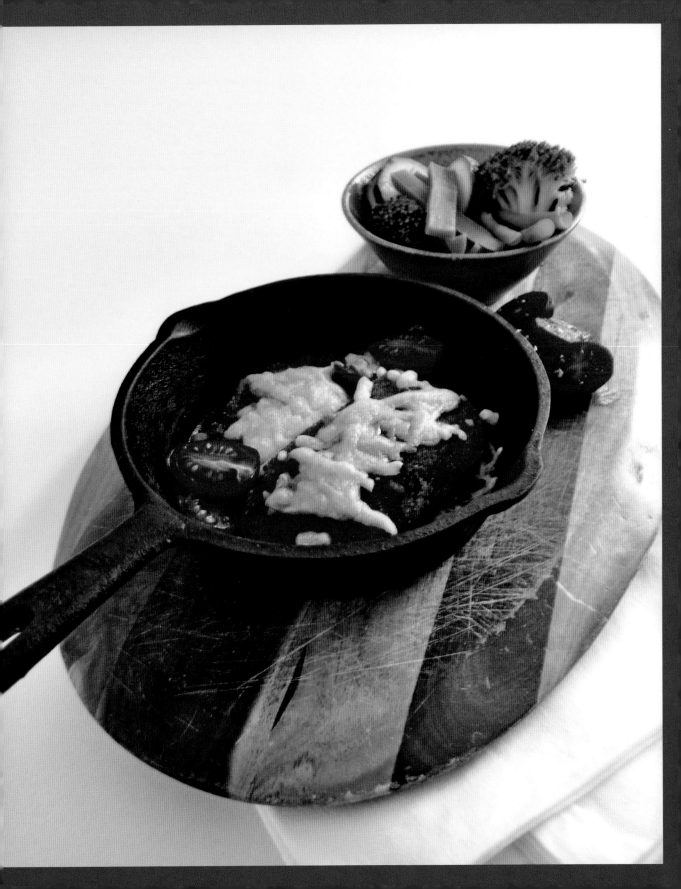

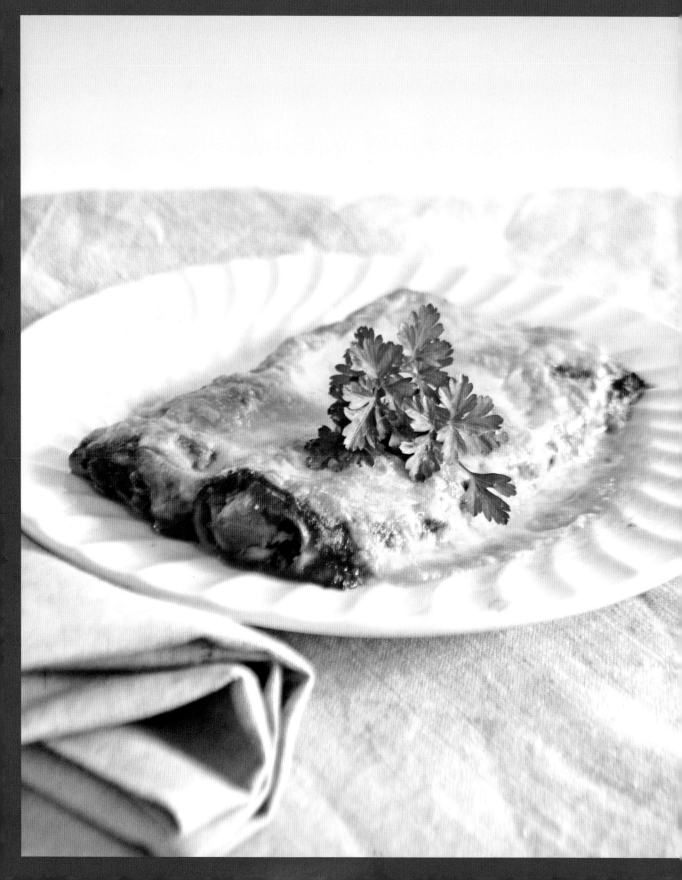

Roasted Pumpkin, Spinach and Ricotta Cannelloni

SERVES TWO ADULTS AND TWO CHILDREN
This meal can be prepared during the day, stored in the fridge and baked before dinner. Serve with a fresh garden salad.

250 g (8 oz) packet of chopped frozen spinach (defrosted in the fridge the night before)

500 g (16 oz) ricotta cheese

300 g (10 oz) roasted pumpkin, cubed (leftovers are ideal for this recipe, sweet potato can be used instead if preferred)

Large pinch nutmeg

Soft lasagne sheets (from cold section of supermarket)

500 ml (16 fl oz) passata

1 clove minced garlic

Pinch dried mixed herbs

180 g (6 oz) cheese, grated

1. Preheat oven to 180°C/160°C fan forced (350°F/gas 4).
2. Snip the corner off the spinach bag and squeeze out excess moisture.
3. Mix the spinach with ricotta cheese until well combined.
4. Add 200 g (6 oz) of the diced pumpkin and nutmeg and fold through gently. Set aside.
5. Lay out 8–10 lasagne sheets on a clean bench that are approximately 16x11 cm (6x4 in) and brush with water on both sides.
6. Spoon out ricotta mixture evenly along the long edge of each sheet until all of the mixture is used. Roll up each sheet and place in a large baking dish.
7. In a large jug mash remaining roasted pumpkin, add passata, garlic and herbs, mix well and pour evenly over cannelloni tubes in baking dish.
8. Sprinkle with cheese and bake in oven for 30–40 minutes, when cheese has melted and pasta sheets are soft.
9. Allow to cool slightly before serving.

Folded Salmon Lasagne

SERVES TWO ADULTS AND TWO CHILDREN
A tasty meal with hidden vegetables for fussy eaters.

Sauce

2 medium sized squash
120 g (4 oz) frozen
 cauliflower florets,
 defrosted
½ onion, finely diced
1 clove garlic, minced
250 ml (8 fl oz) milk
1 tablespoon cornflour
 (cornstarch)
60 g (2 oz) grated cheese
60 ml (2 fl oz) fresh lemon
 juice

Lasagne

6 lasagne sheets
3–4 salmon fillets

1. Place raw squash and cauliflower in a small blender or food processor and puree until smooth. Set aside.
2. In a medium sized non-stick saucepan sauté onion and garlic until onion is transparent.
3. Add puree and stir well, bring to boil, turn down to simmer and cover.
4. In a small bowl combine cornflour and a little of the milk to form a smooth paste, gradually add the rest of the milk, stirring well. Add this to the puree mixture and stir through, bring to boil again, turn down and cover, simmering for at least 15 minutes.
5. While sauce is simmering, boil lasagne sheets in a large saucepan of water, once just *al dente*, remove from heat, do not cover.
6. Grill or fry salmon fillets as desired. Set aside.
7. Stir sauce well and add cheese and lemon juice.
8. Plate lasagne by placing a spoonful of sauce on each plate, followed by a sheet or two of lasagne, another dollop of sauce and the salmon fillet. Fold lasagne sheet over the salmon fillet and finish with another generous spoonful of sauce and grated parmesan cheese. Serve with steamed greens.

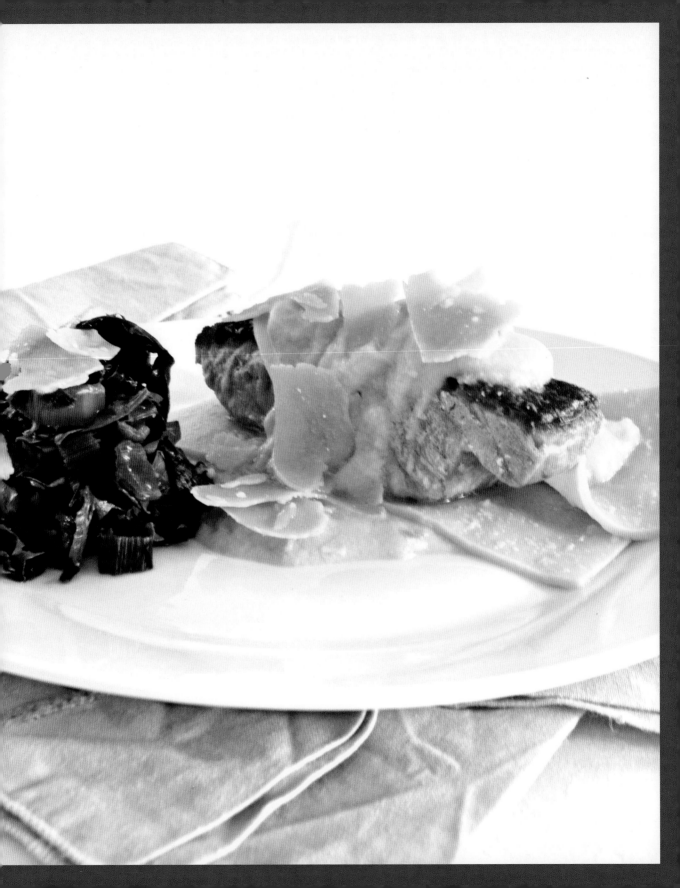

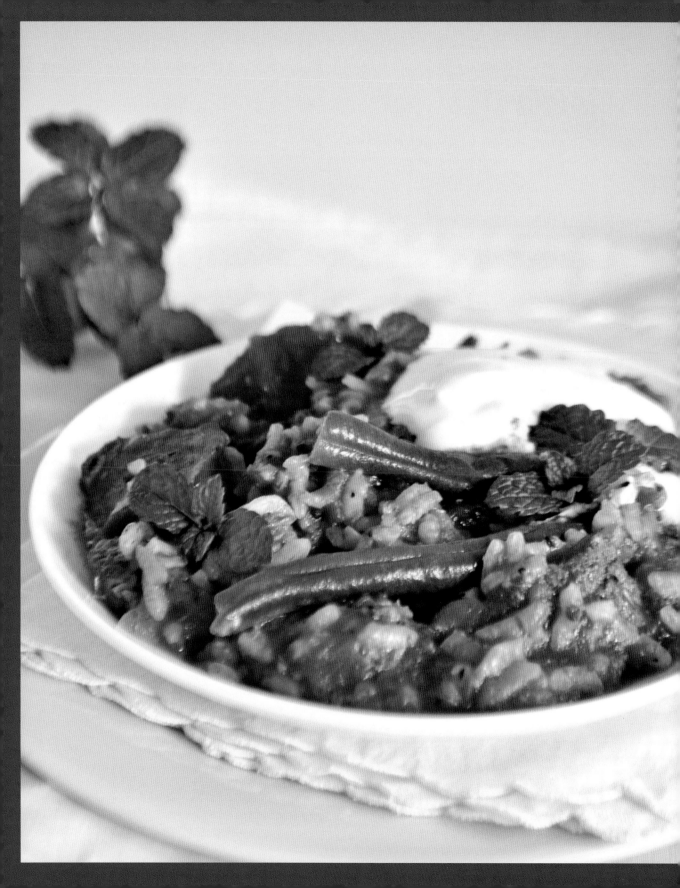

Lovely Leftovers Risotto

SERVES TWO ADULTS AND TWO TODDLERS

Cooking time and amount of water needed may vary depending on type of rice cooker. It is recommended the first time this dish is prepared to check the risotto consistency after 15 minutes of cooking to see if the quantity of water is sufficient. Add more water if necessary.

A quick and nutritious meal using leftovers. Roasted beef can also be used with a pinch of dried oregano instead of thyme, and a handful of halved cherry tomatoes on top in place of the yogurt.

200–250 g (8 oz) leftover roast lamb, diced roughly
200–250 g (8 oz) leftover roasted sweet potato and/or roasted pumpkin diced
100–150 g (4 oz) leftover steamed greens or frozen peas
1 roasted onion
150 g (5 oz) arborio rice
650 ml (21 fl oz) water
1 teaspoon vegetable spread (yeast extract) or similar
¼ lemon with skin on
pinch dried thyme
3 tablespoons Greek style yogurt
Mint leaves to garnish

1. Roughly dice the lamb, sweet potato, pumpkin, greens and onion.
2. Place into rice cooker with rice, water, vegetable spread, lemon and thyme and mix well.
3. Place lid on rice cooker and turn on to the cook setting.
4. Once cooked remove the lemon, serve into bowls and top with yogurt and fresh mint leaves.

No Chop No Prep Risotto

SERVES TWO ADULTS AND TWO TODDLERS

Cooking time and amount of water needed may vary depending on type of rice cooker. It is recommended the first time this dish is prepared to check risotto consistency after 15 minutes of cooking to see if the quantity of water is sufficient. Add more water if necessary.

Serve with fresh herbs or a slice of lemon and a side salad. Add a tablespoon of pesto for an easy alternative. The perfect easy meal after a busy day at work!

250 g (8 oz) packet of chopped frozen spinach (defrosted in the fridge the night before)
150 g (5 oz) arborio rice
500 ml (16 fl oz) water (or chicken stock if preferred)
200 g (7 oz) sliced mushrooms, washed
250 g (8 oz) diced chicken
40 g (1 oz) cheese, grated
2 tablespoons Greek style yogurt
90 ml (3 fl oz) milk

1. Snip the corner off the spinach bag and squeeze out excess moisture.
2. Place spinach, rice, water, mushrooms and chicken in rice cooker and mix well.
3. Place lid on rice cooker and turn on to cook setting.
4. Once cooked, stir through grated cheese, yogurt and the amount of milk you like to achieve desired consistency.

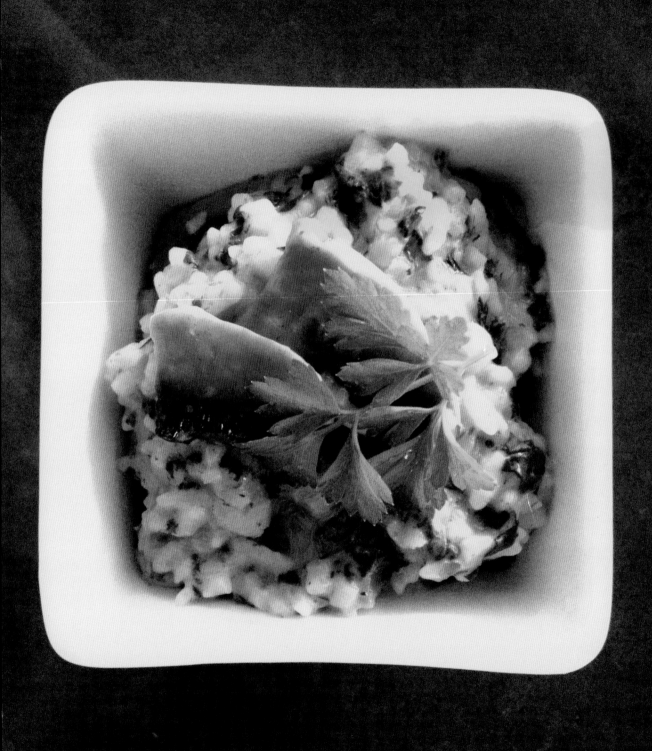

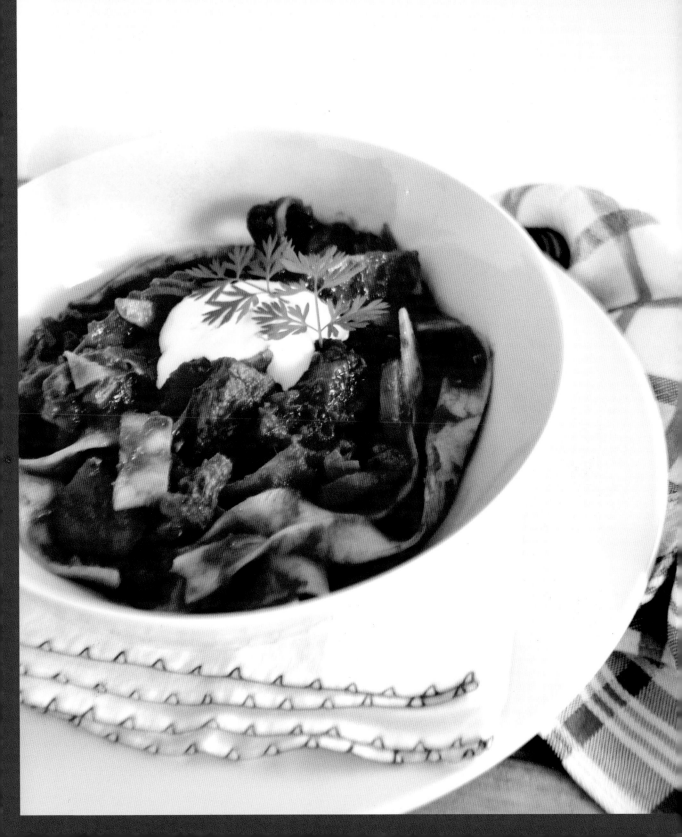

Beef Ragout with Fettuccini

THIS RECIPE IS A BULK DISH THAT SERVES TWO ADULTS AND TWO CHILDREN FOR TWO NIGHTS
Simply freeze half and reheat with some fresh pasta for an easy dinner another night. Serve with a dollop of Greek style yogurt on top of your favorite pasta.

400–500 g (13 oz) chuck or braising steak, diced roughly

1 onion diced

1 clove of garlic, minced or finely chopped

2 large carrots, sliced thinly

1 celery stick, diced small

250 g (8 oz) pumpkin, peeled and cubed

1 heaped teaspoon vegetable spread (yeast extract) or similar

1 dessertspoon dried mixed herbs (or mixed herbs)

50g (1½ oz) red lentils

½ lemon with peel left on

500ml (16 fl oz) passata

500ml (16 fl oz) water

1. Brown steak in a large non-stick frypan or large non-stick saucepan.
2. Add onion and garlic and fry until onion is transparent.
3. Add balance of ingredients, bring to boil then turn down heat, cover and simmer on low for at least 2½ hours. The longer this cooks the more tender the meat becomes and the more flavorsome the dish will be.
4. Remove lid, remove lemon, and using a potato masher, gently mash the mixture to break up the steak and mash the pumpkin. Simmer for another 30–60 minutes, until sauce has reduced and consistency is thick and rich.

A slow cooker or multi-cooker can also be used for this recipe, ensure steam vent is left open during cooking. If you have a slow cooker with a timer, all ingredients can be placed in at once the night before and timer set the next morning before going to work. Skipping the browning step just makes the dish lose a little flavor, but it is still very tasty.

Pork and Apple Terrine

125 g (4 oz) chopped frozen
spinach (defrosted in the
fridge the night before)
500 g (16 oz) pork mince
½ small onion, finely diced
1 clove of garlic minced or
finely chopped
½ red apple peeled, cored
and grated
1 teaspoon allspice
1 egg whisked lightly
45 g (1½ oz) organic
sultanas
½ apple, cored and sliced
thinly

1. Preheat oven to 140°C/160°C fan forced (325°F/gas 3) and line a loaf tin with baking paper.
2. Pat excess moisture from spinach with paper towels, set aside on a clean paper towel.
3. In a large bowl mix mince, onion, garlic, grated apple, allspice and egg with hands to ensure well combined.
4. Spread apple slices in an overlapping fashion on the bottom of the loaf tin. (This will become the decorative topping once the terrine is cooled and flipped upside-down.)
5. Spread half on the mince mixture over the apple to evenly and firmly cover the bottom of the loaf tin.
6. Spread the spinach and sultanas over the mince evenly.
7. Spread remainder of mince evenly and firmly with the back of a dessert spoon.
8. Cover with foil and place in a baking try half filled with boiling water in oven for 2 hours.
9. Remove from oven and cool. Place in fridge overnight with another weighted loaf tin on top. (Three 440 g (14 oz) tins fit in a loaf tin well to weigh it down.)
10. Serve cold the next day with salad for lunch or dinner. This also makes a healthy lunchbox snack.

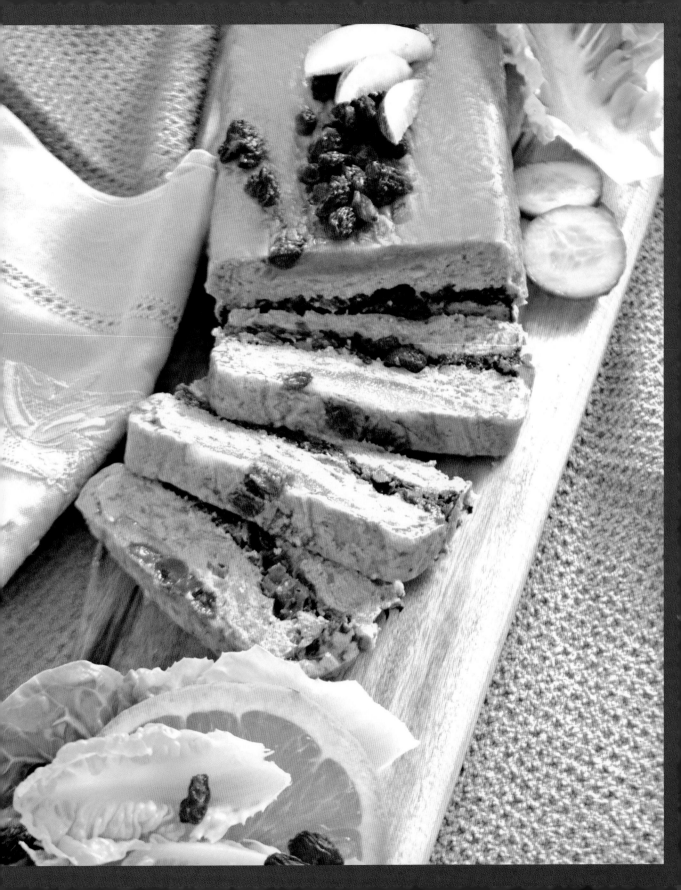

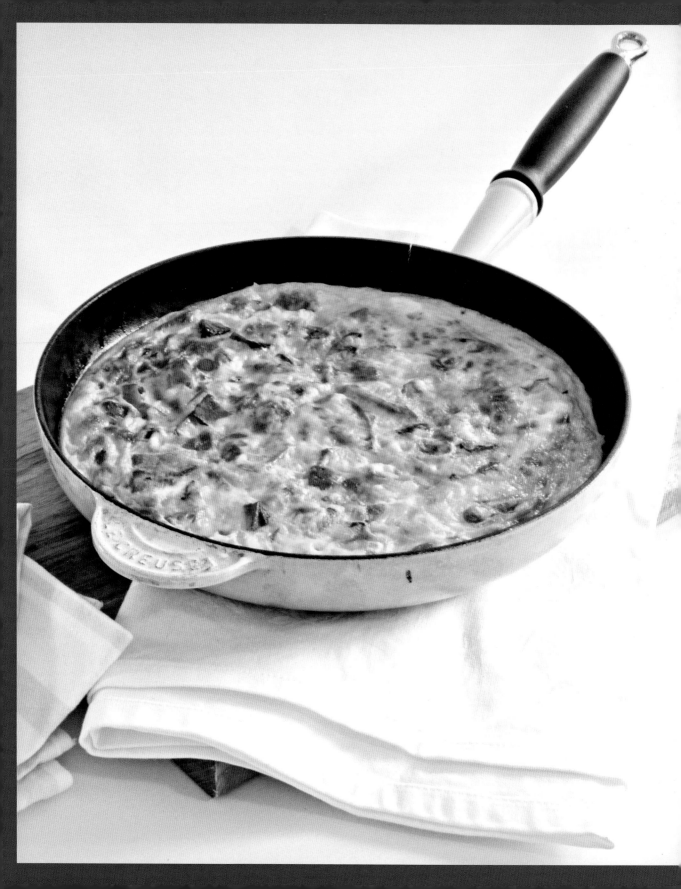

Frittata

SERVES TWO ADULTS AND TWO CHILDREN

Serve with a garden salad for dinner, or cold the next day for lunch.

1 onion finely diced
1 clove of garlic, minced or
   finely chopped
200 g (6½ oz) rindless
   bacon, diced (organic is
   preferred if budget allows,
   or pork fillet is a good
   substitute)
200 g (6½ oz) mushrooms,
   sliced
1 zucchini (courgette),
   grated
5 eggs
130 g (4 oz) Greek style
   yogurt
125 ml (4 fl oz) milk
80 g (2 oz) cheese, grated
140 g (4⅔ oz) frozen corn
   kernels
Tomato for garnish

1. In a large, deep non-stick, ovenproof fry pan, fry onion until transparent.
2. Add garlic and bacon and fry over a high heat until bacon is cooked through.
3. Add mushrooms and zucchini (courgette), sauté, then simmer for 10–15 minutes uncovered until liquid has evaporated.
4. While the mushrooms and zucchini (courgette) is cooking, in a medium mixing bowl whisk eggs, yogurt, milk and half of the cheese until well combined. Set aside.
5. Once the moisture has evaporated form the frypan, add corn kernels and stir through evenly.
6. Pre-heat oven grill to a high setting.
7. Turn heat down in frypan to medium and spread mixture evenly in pan. Slowly pour in egg mixture, cover and simmer gently for approximately 10 minutes or until the bottom of the mixture is cooked and only the top third is runny.
8. Sprinkle cheese and tomato on top of frittata and grill until cooked through and golden brown.

Easy Cheesy Quiche

SERVES THREE ADULTS AND TWO TODDLERS

Serve with a garden salad and fresh bread rolls. Substitute spinach and pumpkin with corn kernels and bacon, or leftover roasted vegetables for easy alternatives. Leftovers can be eaten cold the next day.

This dish can be prepared during the day, stored in the fridge and popped in the oven before dinner.

250 g (8 oz) packet of chopped frozen spinach (defrosted in the fridge the night before)
½ small onion, finely diced
100 g (3⅓ oz) raw pumpkin, grated
5 eggs
80 g (2 ½ oz) cheese, grated
80 g (2 ½ oz) Danish fetta cheese, crumbled roughly
125 ml (4 fl oz) milk

1. Preheat oven to 180°C/160°C fan forced (350°F/gas 4) and line a pie dish with baking paper.
2. Snip the corner off the spinach bag and squeeze out excess moisture.
3. Mix all ingredients, pour into lined pie dish and bake for approximately 1 hour or until firm and golden.
4. Allow to cool slightly before serving.

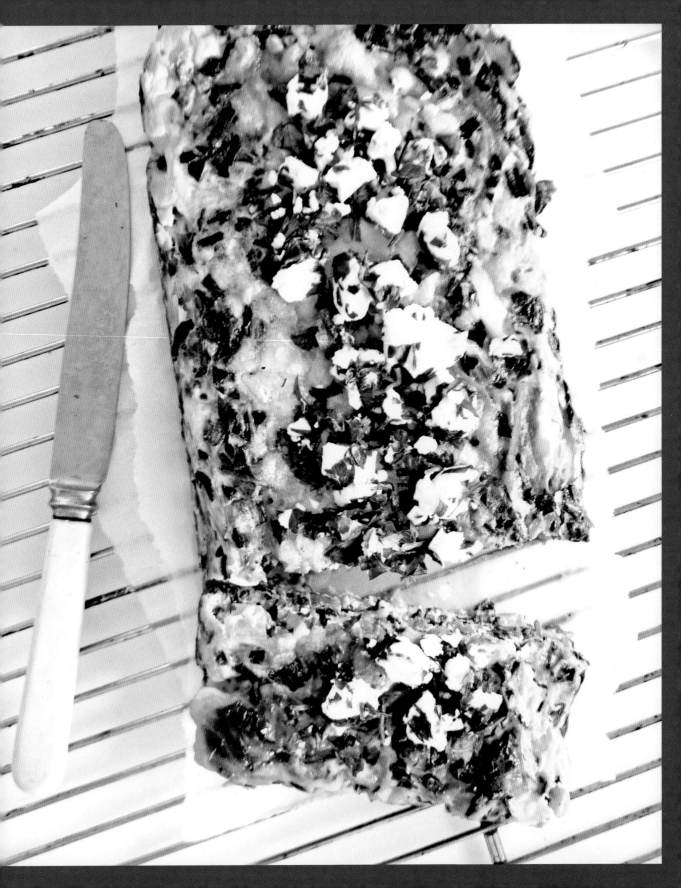

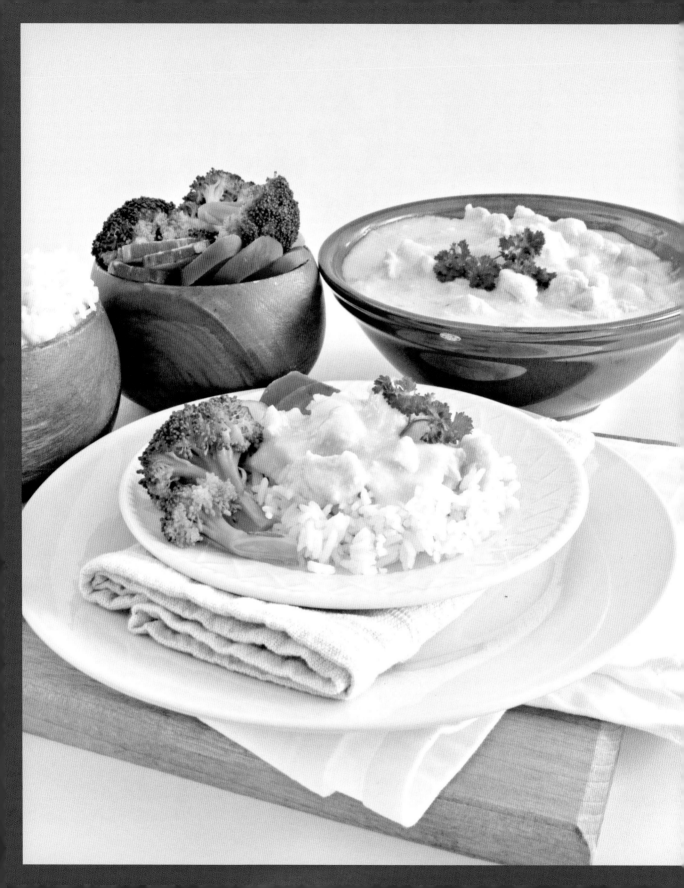

Cauliflower and Cheese Chicken

SERVES TWO ADULTS AND TWO TODDLERS

A good dish for children who are going through their 'only eating white things' stage. Serve with steamed rice and vegetables or salad.

330 g (11 oz) frozen cauliflower (defrosted in the fridge the night before)

250 ml (8 fl oz) water

1 onion, finely diced

500 g (16 oz) chicken breast or thigh fillet, diced

1 clove of garlic, minced or finely chopped

2 tablespoons cornflour (cornstarch)

125 ml (4 fl oz) milk

40 g (1 oz) cheese, grated

1. Puree cauliflower and water in a food processor. Set aside.
2. In a large deep non-stick fry pan, fry over a medium-high heat, onion and chicken until onion is transparent and chicken is slightly brown.
3. Add garlic and fry for another few minutes. Set aside.
4. In a small cup mix cornflour and a little of the milk to make a paste, gradually add the rest of the milk mixing well.
5. Add the cornflour and milk mixture to the frypan and stir in well.
6. Bring to boil whilst stirring continuously, turn down to a simmer and stir for another 5–10 minutes until thick and silky.
7. Add grated cheese and stir through. More cheese can be added if desired.

Lamb Koftas and Cous Cous Salad

MAKES 8–10 SMALL SERVES

A great lunch to share with friends or fun dinner for the family.

Cous Cous Salad

200 g (7 oz) sweet potato steamed and
  diced (leftovers of freshly steamed)
70 g (2⅓ oz) wholemeal cous cous
125 ml (4 fl oz) boiling water
3 tablespoons roughly chopped mint leaves
3 tablespoons roughly chopped parsley
  leaves
juice of ½ lemon
1 tablespoon finely diced onion
2 tablespoons sultanas
2 tablespoons flaked almonds

Koftas

500 g (17 oz) lean lamb mince
2 tablespoons finely chopped mint leaves
2 tablespoons finely chopped parsley leaves
1 teaspoon garlic, minced
1 heaped teaspoon ground cumin seeds
1 heaped teaspoon ground coriander seeds

8–10 paddle pop sticks or skewers soaked
  in water overnight
8–10 small pita pocket breads (to serve)
125 ml (4 fl oz) Greek style yogurt and
  lemon wedges (to serve)

1. Steam sweet potato and dice into small cubes. Set aside.
2. Place cous cous into a large mixing bowl and pour boiling water over.
3. Once cous cous has absorbed the water, fluff up the mixture with a fork and fold through sweet potato. Place in refrigerator to cool.
4. In a large bowl mix all the kofta ingredients until well combined.
5. Divide mixture into 8-10 portions and mould each portion onto paddle pop sticks, forming a flat oval shape at one end of the stick.
6. Cook in a non-stick frypan or on a BBQ.
7. While koftas are cooking fold remaining cous cous ingredients through the cous cous mixture and return to fridge until serving time.
8. Serve koftas in pita pocket breads with cous cous salad, a dollop of yogurt and a squeeze of fresh lemon.

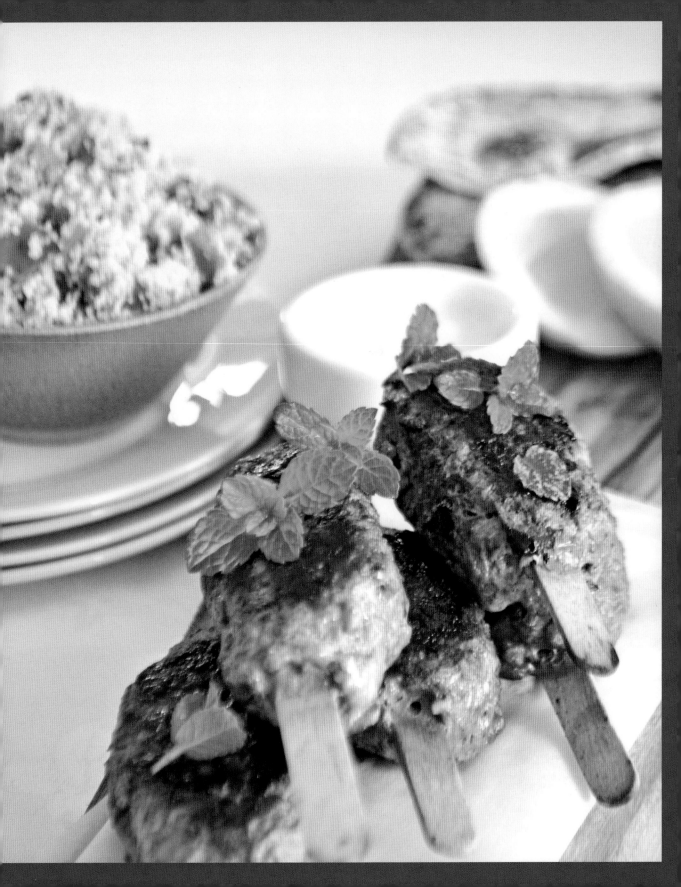

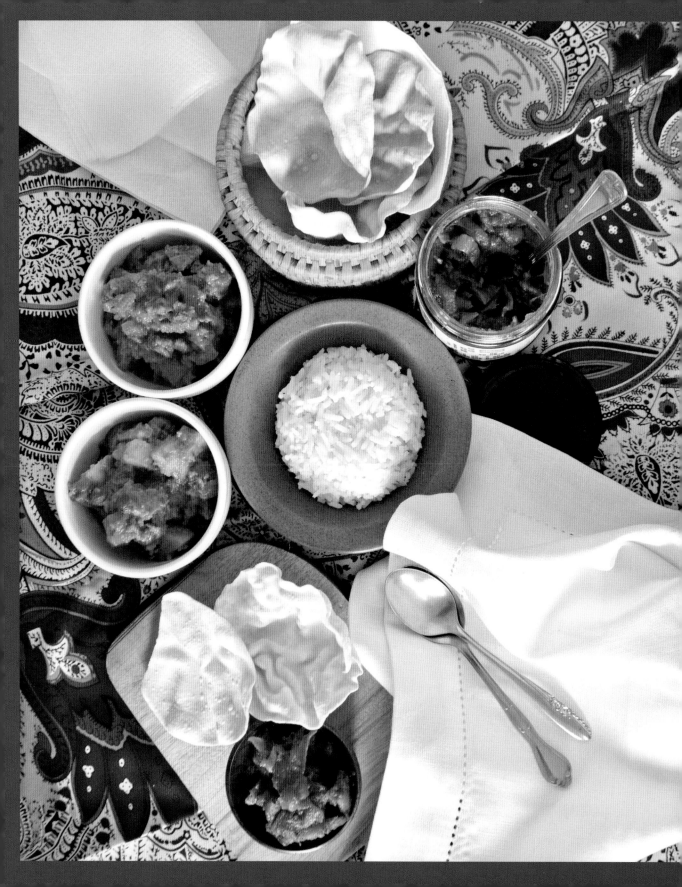

Beginners Curry

Serve with steamed rice, papadums and chutney.

300 g (10 oz) pumpkin diced into 1 cm (½ in) cubes

1 onion, finely diced

1 clove of garlic, minced or finely chopped

2 teaspoon of ground cumin seeds

2 teaspoon of ground coriander seeds

½ teaspoon cayenne pepper

½ teaspoon mustard powder

2 small potatoes diced into 1 cm (½ in) cubes

1 medium sweet potato diced into 1 cm (½ in) cubes

1 red apple cored and diced into 1 cm (½ in) cubes

125 ml (4 fl oz) passata

1 teaspoon vegetable spread (yeast extract) or similar

65 g (2 oz) organic sultanas

125 ml (4 fl oz) water

1 x 400ml (13 fl oz) can coconut milk

400 g (13 oz) beef rump steak diced

1. Puree raw diced pumpkin in a food processor, if the mixture is a little dry add 125 ml (4 fl oz) water. Set aside.
2. In a large deep non-stick fry pan, fry onion, garlic and spices until onion is transparent.
3. Add diced vegetables and apple, fry over a medium heat, turning occasionally for 5 minutes.
4. Add balance of ingredients and stir well.
5. Bring to boil, cover and simmer for 20–30 minutes until potatoes are soft and beef is tender.

Cheeky Chicken Stir Fry

SERVES TWO ADULTS AND TWO TODDLERS

Serve with your favorite noodles or rice. Capsicum (peppers), baby corn, broccoli or Asian greens can be added or substituted if preferred. Rice noodles tend to have the least amount of artificial additives, colors and preservatives, check the ingredients when shopping.

125 ml (4 fl oz) freshly squeezed orange juice

2 tablespoons natural soy sauce (check ingredients to avoid unnecessary chemicals and preservatives)

1 teaspoon honey

225 g (7 oz) finely grated pumpkin (use a zester grater)

1 onion, finely diced

1 clove of garlic, minced or finely chopped

40–500 g (13-16 oz) diced chicken 1 carrot, cut into narrow sticks

A small handful of green beans (15–20) 'topped and tailed'125 ml (4 fl oz) water

1 zucchini (courgette) sliced into thin sticks

A small handful of snow peas (15–20) 'topped and tailed'

1. In a small bowl mix orange juice, soy sauce and honey. Set this orange sauce mix aside.
2. In a large deep non-stick frypan sauté pumpkin and onion until it begins to soften.
3. Add garlic and chicken and fry on a medium-high heat until all sides of chicken cubes are sealed and slightly brown.
4. Add carrot and green beans and water, stir and cover, cook for 2 minutes.
5. Add balance of ingredients, stir and cover, cook for 1 minute.

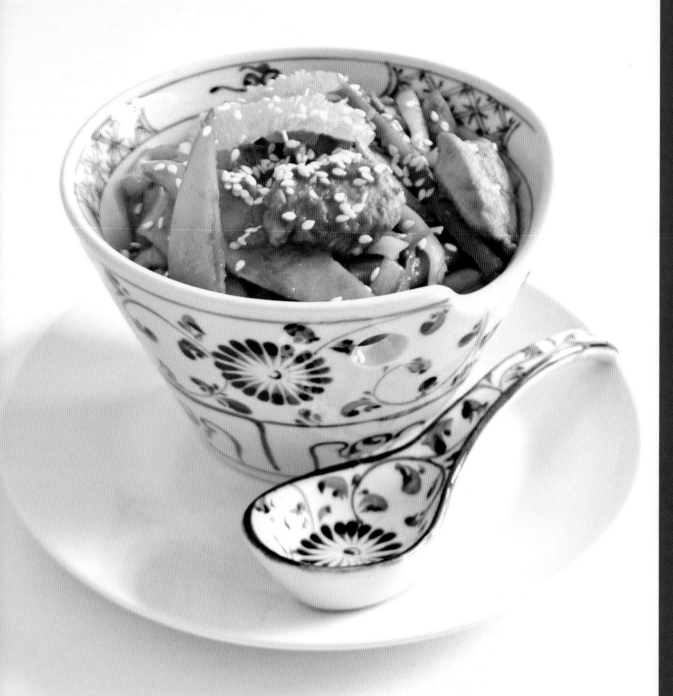

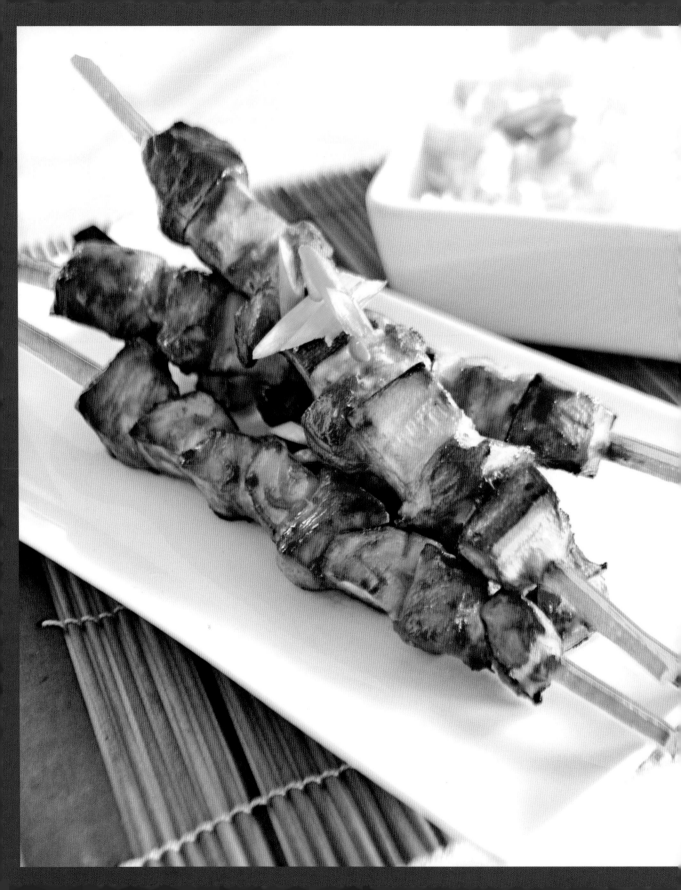

Asian Style Skewers

Serve with rice and steamed vegetables. Skewers can also be made the night before and marinated in the sauce in an airtight container.

1 zucchini (courgette)
220 g (7 oz) diced chicken
8 skewers or disposable
   wooden chopsticks
   soaked in water overnight

Sauce

1 tablespoon sweet chilli
   sauce
1 tablespoon soy sauce
1 tablespoon honey
½ teaspoon garlic, minced
½ teaspoon ginger, minced

1. Cut zucchini into 1 cm (¾ in) slices, and quarter each slice.
2. Fill the skewers alternating between chicken and zucchini cubes. Place skewers on a large tray and set aside.
3. Mix all sauce ingredients in a small bowl and coat the chicken and zucchini with the sauce mixture using a pastry brush until well covered.
4. Grill in oven or fry skewers in a non-stick frypan over a medium heat, turning until all sides are golden brown and chicken is cooked through.

Fried Rice

This is a tasty dish to use leftover rice from the night before. Serve with steamed green vegetables. If desired, shredded chicken or bacon can also be added to the fried rice.

1 onion, diced
1 large carrot, finely diced
1 stick of celery, finely diced
1 clove of garlic, minced or finely chopped
300 g (10 oz) cooked, cold rice
75 g (2 ½ oz) corn kernels (fresh or frozen)
75 g (2 ½ oz) frozen peas
1–3 dessertspoons soy sauce
2 tablespoons honey
4 eggs

1. In a large deep non-stick fry pan, fry over a medium-high heat the onion and carrot for 2 minutes.
2. Add celery and garlic, frying until onion is transparent.
3. Add rice, corn and peas and fry for another few minutes.
4. Add soy sauce (gradually, to taste) and honey and mix through well. Set aside with a lid on to keep warm.
5. In a separate non-stick frypan fry eggs to serve on top of rice.

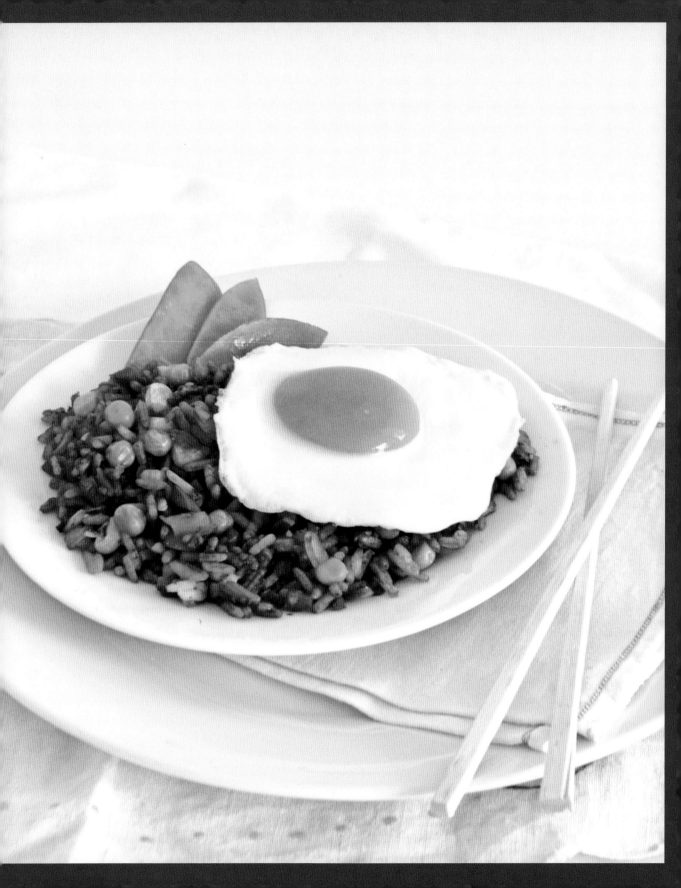

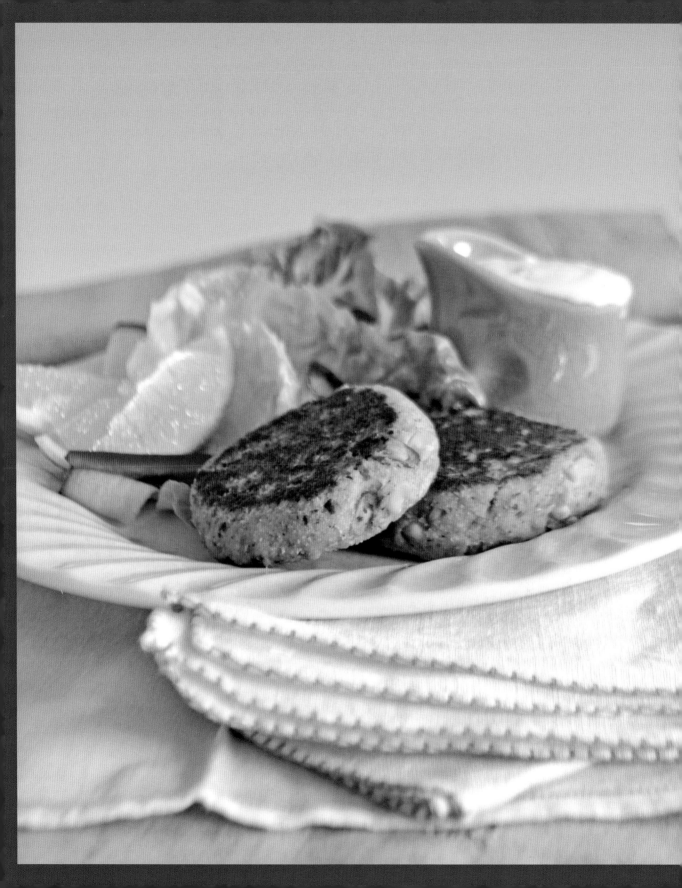

Fish Cakes

MAKES 8 FISH CAKES. SERVES TWO ADULTS AND TWO TODDLERS.

These fish cakes can be refrigerated prior to cooking if prepared in the morning.

An ideal dish for children who are being introduced to fish. Serve with chunky chips (see page 61) and vegetables or salad. These can also be eaten cold the next day.

250 g (8 oz) fresh white fish fillets (frozen and defrosted are fine)
4 slices of wholemeal bread
½ onion
small bunch fresh parsley (or coriander if preferred)
½ teaspoon minced ginger
1 egg
1 tablespoon lemon juice
10–12 green beans, sliced thinly
70 g (2⅓ oz) corn kernels

Dipping Sauce
130g (4oz) Greek style yogurt
¼ clove of garlic, minced or finely chopped
1 tablespoon lemon juice

1. Puree fish, bread, onion, parsley, ginger, egg and lemon juice in a food processor until smooth.
2. Transfer fish mixture into a large mixing bowl and add beans and corn. Mix well.
3. Using a tablespoon, form 5 cm (2 in) balls and slightly flatten between palms of hands to form patties. Place on a large plate.
4. In a large deep non-stick fry pan, fry fish cakes over a medium heat until golden brown on both sides. If the cakes feel soft to touch place a lid on the frypan for a few minutes to ensure the cakes are cooked through and firm.
5. In a small cup mix dipping sauce ingredients together.

Satay Chicken

SERVES TWO ADULTS AND TWO TODDLERS
Serve with steamed rice and vegetables or salad.

½ onion, finely diced
1 clove of garlic, minced or
  finely chopped
1 large carrot, sliced
3 chicken thigh fillets or
  2 breast fillets, diced
90 g (3 oz) pumpkin,
  coarsely grated
125 ml (4 fl oz) water

Sauce
1 tablespoon soy sauce
1 teaspoon vegetable
  spread (yeast extract)
2 tablespoons peanut butter
2 tablespoons honey
60 ml (2 fl oz) boiling water

1. In a large deep non-stick fry pan, fry over a medium-high heat the onion, garlic, carrot and chicken until onion is transparent and chicken is slightly brown.
2. Add grated pumpkin and fry for another few minutes.
3. Add water and cover, simmering for a few minutes to allow pumpkin to soften.
4. In a small cup mix soy sauce, vegetable spread (yeast extract), peanut butter and honey. Add boiling water and whisk with a fork until well combined.
5. Add the sauce mixture to the frypan and stir in well.
6. Bring to boil whilst stirring continuously, turn down to a simmer and stir for another 2–5 minutes.

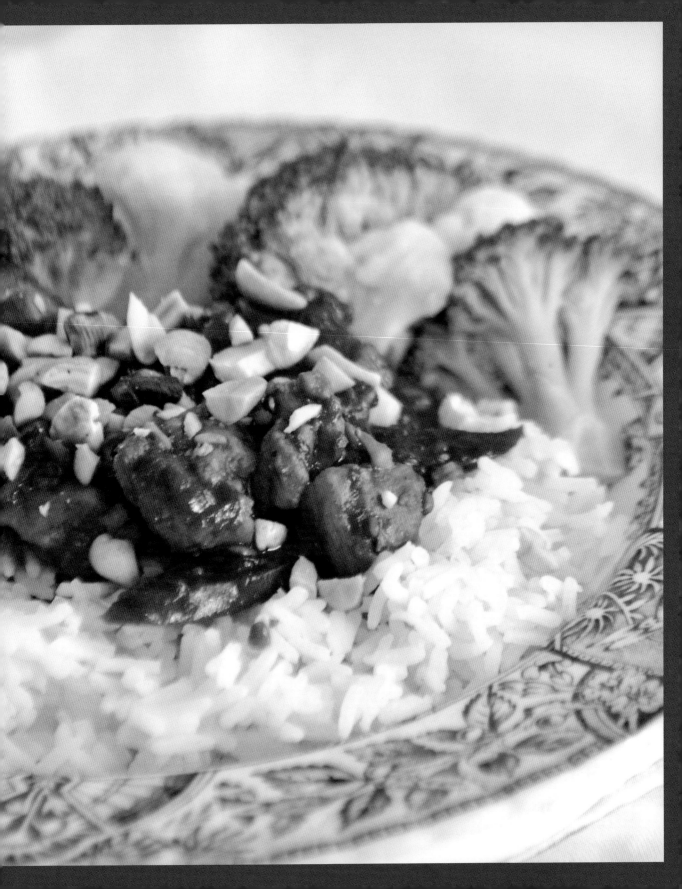

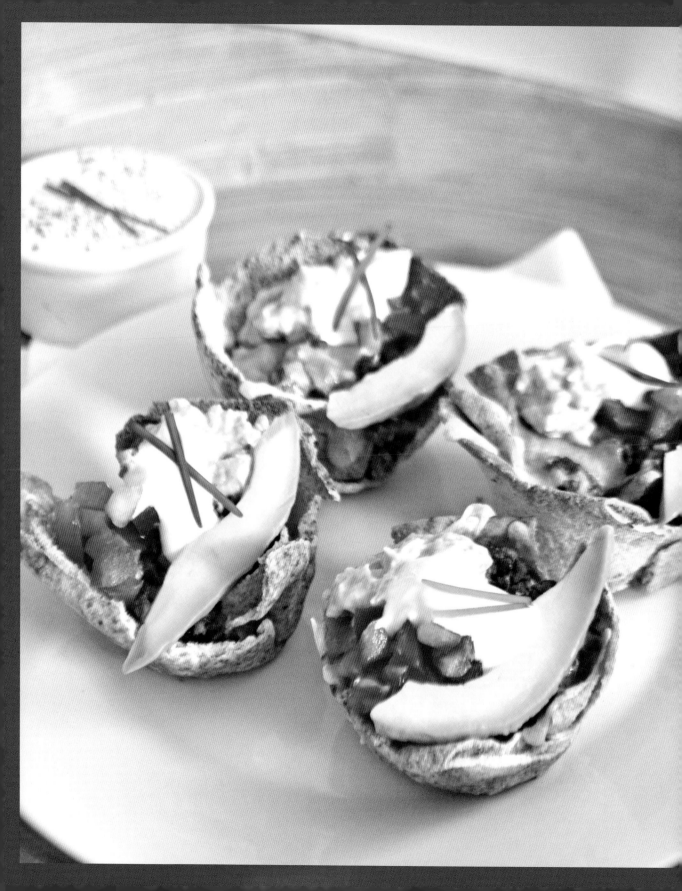

Healthy Nacho Cups

SERVES TWO ADULTS AND TWO TODDLERS
Mince can be doubled and half frozen for a future easy meal.

Chip Cups
3 large wholemeal pita or
  Lebanese breads

Guacamole
1 large avocado
1 teaspoon freshly
  squeezed lemon juice
1 heaped dessertspoon
  Greek style yogurt

Salsa
2 large ripe tomatoes
¼ red capsicum (pepper)
  (optional)

Mince
1 onion, finely diced
1 clove of garlic, minced or
  finely chopped
250 g (8 oz) beef mince
2 teaspoons of ground
  cumin seeds
125 g (4 oz) of chopped frozen
  spinach (defrosted in the
  fridge the night before)
125 ml (4 fl oz) passata
1 teaspoon vegetable spread
  (yeast extract)
260 g (8 ¼ oz) Greek style
  yogurt
80 g (2 ½ oz) cheese, grated

Chip Cups
1. Preheat oven to 180°C/160°C fan forced (350°F/gas 4). Line a large muffin tray with baking paper or muffin papers.
2. Cut wholemeal pita or Lebanese breads into quarters with kitchen scissors. Press firmly into lined muffin tray to form individual cups and bake for 5-10 minutes until crunchy but not brown. Set aside.
3. If the bread pops out of tray simply weigh down with pastry weights or small ramekins.

Guacamole
1. Mash all ingredients together and store in fridge until serving.

Salsa
1. Dice tomatoes and capsicum and place in a small bowl and store in fridge until serving.

Mince and Nachos
1. In a large deep non-stick fry pan, fry onion until transparent.
2. Add garlic, mince and spices, stir and fry over a high heat until mince is well browned.
3. Add spinach, half of passata and vegetable spread, bring to boil, then simmer for 5-10 minutes uncovered until sauce has reduced.
4. Spoon mince mixture into chip cups in muffin tray.
5. Pour balance of passata over mince, followed by half of yogurt and top with cheese.
6. Place under grill or at the top of hot oven until cheese is melted and golden.
7. Serve with remaining cold yogurt, salsa and guacamole.

Chicken Enchiladas

SERVES TWO ADULTS AND TWO CHILDREN

Chicken mixture can be doubled and half frozen for a future easy meal. Enchiladas can also be prepared the night or morning before, refrigerated, and baked in the oven at 180°C/160°C fan forced (350°F/gas 4) for 30 minutes, or until piping hot.

½ onion, finely diced

1 clove of garlic, minced or finely chopped

1 teaspoon of ground cumin seeds

1 large chicken breast or 2 thigh fillets, diced into small pieces

200g (7oz) tinned cannellini beans, drained

45 g (1.5 oz) chopped frozen spinach (defrosted in the fridge the night before)

70 g (2⅓ oz) frozen corn kernels

180 ml (6 fl oz) passata

4 wholemeal wraps or mountain bread wraps (check ingredients for least amount of additives and preservatives)

90 g (3 oz) Greek style yogurt

40 g (1 oz) cheese, grated

1. In a large, deep non-stick fry pan, fry onion until transparent.
2. Add garlic, cumin and chicken, stir and fry over a high heat until chicken is well browned.
3. Add cannellini beans, spinach, corn, ¾ of passata and bring to boil, then simmer for 5–10 minutes uncovered until sauce has reduced.
4. Lay out 4 wraps on kitchen bench and spoon chicken mixture along one end of each wrap. If your children are younger you may want to spoon smaller quantities into their wraps.
5. Roll up wraps and place in a baking dish.
6. Pour balance of passata over wraps followed by yogurt, then top with cheese.
7. Place under grill or at the top of hot oven until cheese is melted and golden.
8. Serve with a garden salad and steamed rice.

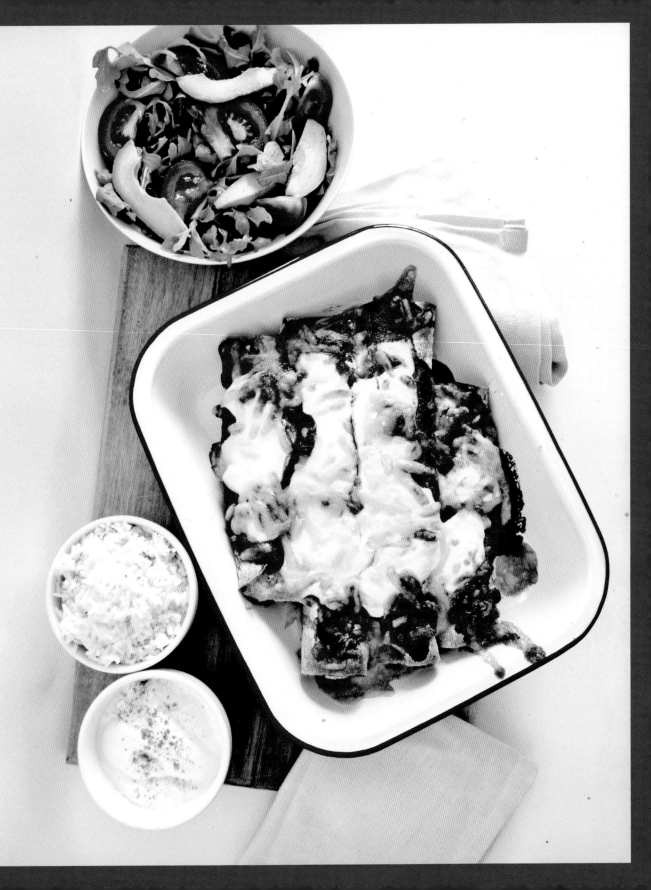

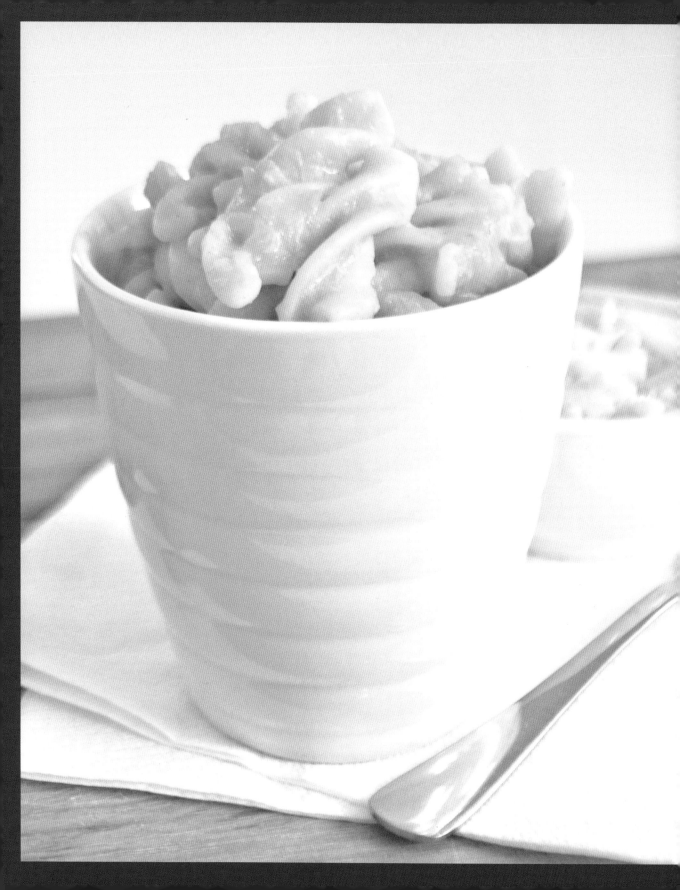

One Pot Cheesy Spirals

A great dinner served with a garden salad, or an easy weekend lunch snack.

180–270 g (6–9 oz) pasta spirals (depending on family size)

½ onion

1 clove garlic

300 g (10 oz) diced pumpkin (small cubes)

125 ml (4 fl oz) water

70 g (2⅓ oz) corn kernels (fresh or frozen)

125 ml (4 fl oz) milk

120 g (3 ½ oz) cheese, grated

1. In a large non-stick saucepan boil pasta as per directions on packaging.
2. While pasta is cooking, finely chop onion, garlic and pumpkin, set aside.
3. Place corn and milk in a small food processor and blend until smooth, set aside.
4. Once pasta is cooked, drain and cover to keep warm.
5. Place onion and garlic in saucepan and fry until onion has softened and is transparent. If you do not have a non-stick saucepan, add a little olive oil to fry with.
6. Add pumpkin and water and bring to boil, cover and simmer until pumpkin is soft and begins to fall apart.
7. Add corn and milk mixture and stir through, simmer for a couple of minutes.
8. Add ¾ of grated cheese and mix through well, add more to taste if necessary.
9. Fold the rest of the cheese through pasta and serve.

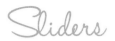
Sliders

SERVES TWO ADULTS AND TWO CHILDREN WITH ENOUGH PATTIES TO FREEZE (UNCOOKED) FOR
ANOTHER NIGHT.

Beef Pattie

500 g (17 oz) fresh lean beef
   mince
1 egg
1 small onion, finely diced
½ small zucchini (courgette)
   grated finely (use a zester
   grater)
70 g (2⅓ oz) pumpkin
   grated finely (use a zester
   grater)
1 heaped tablespoon finely
   chopped celery leaf or
   parsley
1 slice of wholemeal bread,
   chopped finely

Slider Roll and Filling

6 small slices of cheese
6 wholemeal dinner rolls
Handful of baby spinach
   leaves, washed
6 slices of tomato
1 raw baby beetroot, peeled
   and grated
Good quality tomato sauce
   or mayonnaise

1. Mix all ingredients for beef patties thoroughly, using
   a tablespoon form 12 balls and flatten into patties
   between palms of hands. Make 6 patties for one meal
   for 2 adults and 2 children, the other 6 can be frozen in
   an airtight container with greaseproof paper between
   them for another night, as long as the mince hasn't
   been frozen previously.
2. In a non-stick frypan, cook patties over a medium
   heat until well browned on one side, flip patties over
   and place a cheese slice on the cooked side of each to
   enable it to melt slightly.
3. Assemble sliders with spinach leaves, tomato, beetroot
   and beef pattie, topping with a good quality tomato
   sauce or mayonnaise.
4. Serve with chunky chips (see page 61).

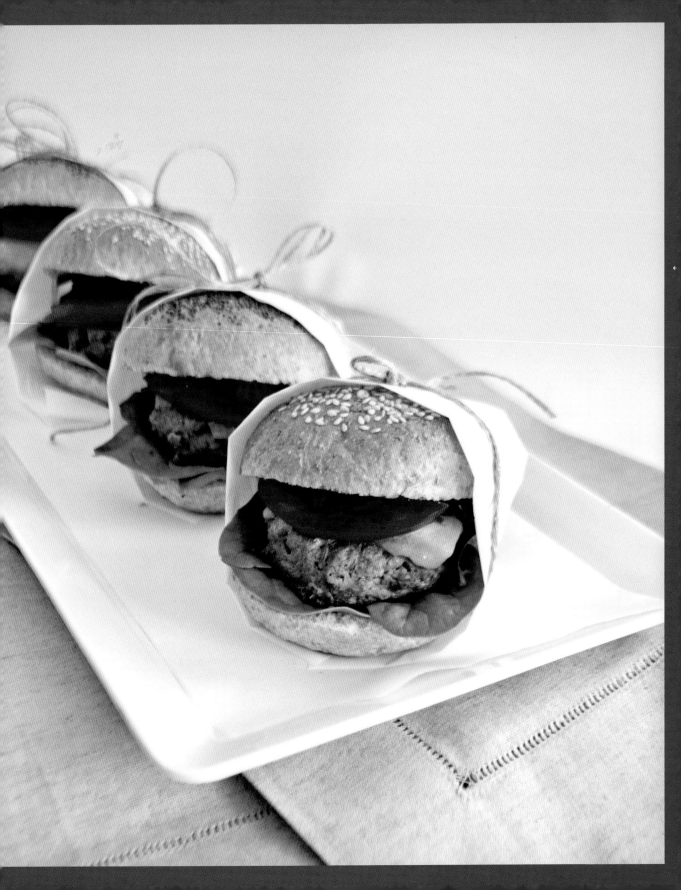

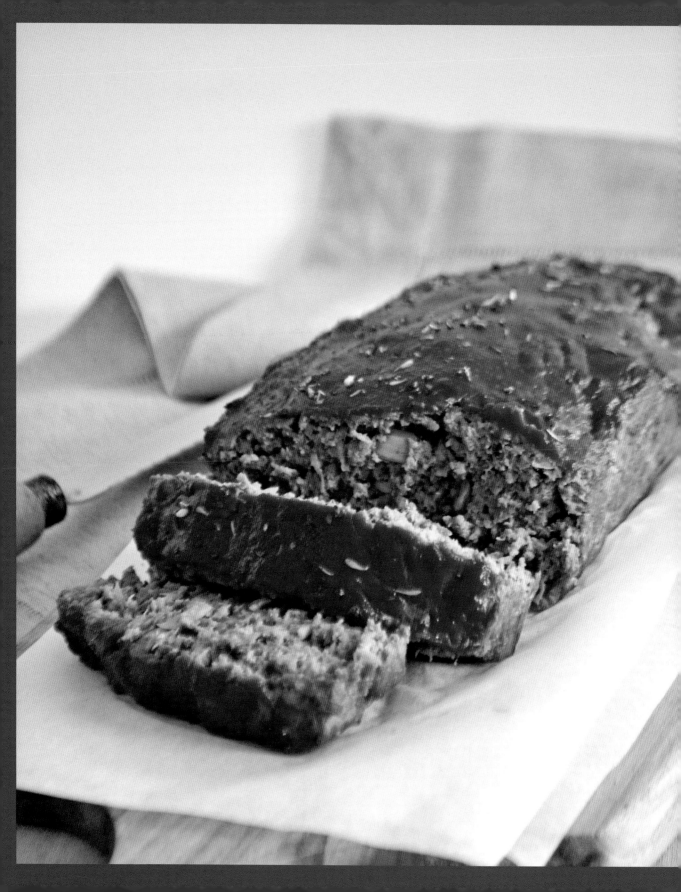

Mischievous Meatloaf

SERVES A FAMILY OF SIX, OR A FAMILY OF FOUR WITH LEFTOVERS FOR LUNCH THE NEXT DAY.
Serve warm with mashed potato and steamed vegetables for dinner, or cold on sandwiches or with salad for lunch the next day. Meatloaf also makes a great lunchbox snack. This meatloaf can also be frozen and reheated for an easy midweek meal.

3 slices wholemeal bread
1 large carrot, grated finely (use zester grater)
90 g (3 oz) frozen spinach (defrosted the night before)
1 onion, finely diced
1 clove of garlic, minced or finely chopped
1 egg, whisked lightly
250 ml (8 fl oz) passata
2 teaspoons dried herbs
500 g (17 oz) beef mince

1. Preheat oven to 180°C/160°C fan forced (350°F/gas 4) and line a loaf tin with baking paper.
2. Toast bread and cut into ½ cm (¼ in) squares and place in a large mixing bowl.
3. Add grated carrot, spinach, diced onion, garlic, egg, half of the passata, 1 teaspoon of the herbs and mix until well combined.
4. Add mince and mix thoroughly with hands until toast is soft and combined evenly into the mixture.
5. Place the mince mixture into loaf tin and press down firmly. Pour the balance of the passata over the top and sprinkle the remaining herbs over the top.
6. Bake for 50 minutes, remove from oven and cover with foil and rest for 10 minutes.

Tuna and Potato Croquette Fingers

MAKES 18–20 FINGERS

Serve warm with salad or steamed vegetables and a wedge of lemon for dinner. These crunchy fingers can be pre-made the morning or night before and stored in the refrigerator and baked just before dinner.

Crumb

2 slices of wholemeal bread with crusts on
10 g (3.5 oz) parmesan cheese
1 egg white, whisked lightly

Filling

250 g (8 oz) potatoes (2 medium potatoes)
185 g (6 oz) canned tuna in springwater, drained well
60 g (2 oz) diced capsicum (peppers) (red and yellow are a great color combination, corn kernels or peas can also be used)
Zest of ½ lemon
60 ml (2 fl oz) lemon juice
1 egg yolk
4 tablespoons cornflour (cornstarch)

1. Preheat oven to 180°C/160°C fan forced (350°F/gas 4) and line a large baking tray with baking paper.
2. Toast bread and place with parmesan cheese into a small blender or food processor. Process to a fine crumb. Pour onto a flat plate and set aside.
3. Peel, quarter and boil potatoes until soft. Drain well and mash.
4. In a large mixing bowl combine mashed potato with balance of filling ingredients until thoroughly combined.
5. Using a level dessertspoon, form potato mixture into a sausage-like shapes between the palms of your hands and press into breadcrumb mixture turning gently and pressing down on sides to crumb well and form a fish finger shape.
6. Place croquette fingers onto a baking tray. Once all of the mixture in shaped and crumbed use a pastry brush to roughly dab each side with whisked egg.
7. Bake for 15 minutes, turn over and bake for a further 15–20 minutes, or until brown and crunchy.

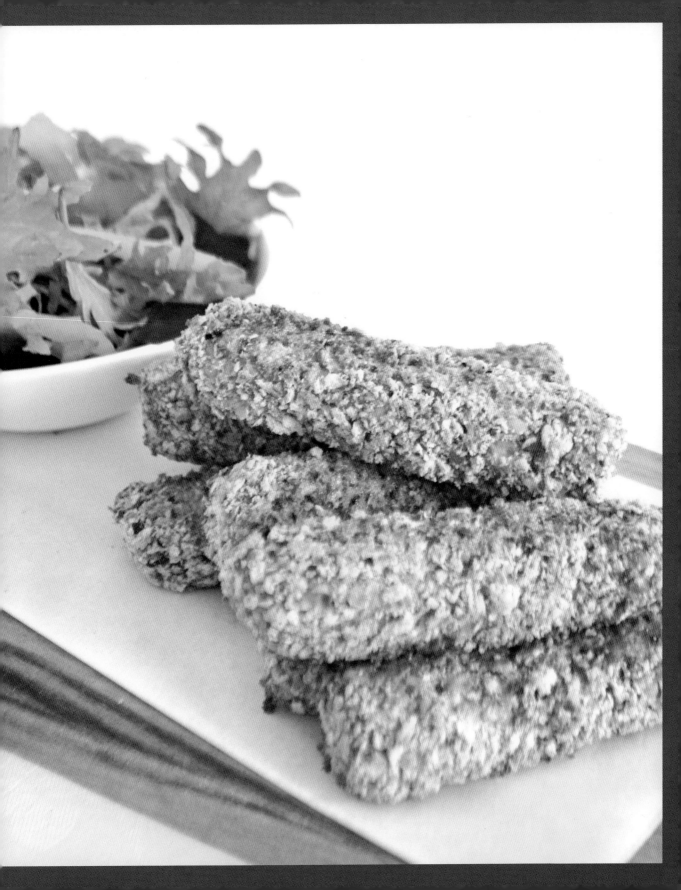

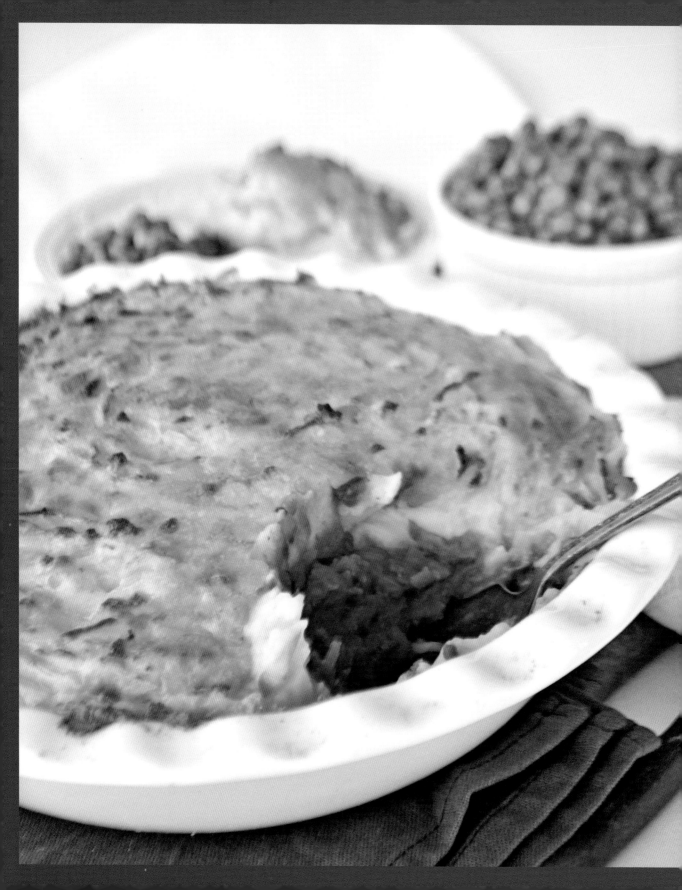

Shepherd's Pie

SERVES TWO–THREE ADULTS AND TWO CHILDREN

Serve with steamed green vegetables or a garden salad. Carrot and/or zucchini (courgette) can be substituted with capsicum (peppers) or squash if preferred.

Filling

500 g (16 oz) beef mince (or half beef, half pork)

1 onion, diced

2 cloves of garlic, minced or finely chopped

1 large carrot, grated coarsely

1 large zucchini (courgette), grated coarsely

1 heaped teaspoon vegetable spread (yeast extract) or similar

1 dessertspoon mixed herbs

75 g (2 ½ oz) red lentils

375 ml (12 fl oz) passata

500 ml (20 fl oz) water

Topping

4 large potatoes peeled and cubed

200 g (7 oz) tinned cannellini beans, drained

4 tablespoons milk

40 g (1 oz) cheese, grated

1. Brown mince and onion in a large non-stick frypan or large non-stick saucepan.
2. Add garlic, carrot, zucchini, vegetable spread (yeast extract) and fry for 5 minutes, turning frequently until vegetables begin to soften.
3. Add balance of filling ingredients, bring to boil then turn down heat, cover and simmer for at least 30 minutes, or until lentils are soft and filling mixture is thick. The pan can be uncovered after 30 minutes to allow faster reduction and thickening.
4. While filling is simmering, boil potatoes until soft, drain and return to saucepan.
5. Puree drained beans and milk to form a smooth paste.
6. Add puree to potatoes in saucepan and mash well. Add a little more milk if necessary.
7. Pour filling into a pie dish and top with potato mixture and lastly grated cheese.
8. Place under grill or at the top of hot oven until cheese is melted and potato topping is golden.

Chipolata and Tomato Casserole

SERVES TWO ADULTS AND TWO TODDLERS
Serve with steamed rice and vegetables or salad.

180 g (6 oz) diced pumpkin
2 medium carrots, chopped
   roughly
375 ml (12 fl oz) passata
1 onion, finely diced
500 g (17 oz) chipolata
   sausages (organic or
   preservative free is best,
   beef, chicken or pork)
1 clove of garlic, minced or
   finely chopped
2 small potatoes, diced into
   1 cm ($^1/_2$ in) cubes
1 medium sweet potato,
   diced into 1 cm ($^1/_2$ in)
   cubes
250 ml (5 fl oz) water
1 teaspoon of dried mixed
   herbs

1. Puree raw diced pumpkin and carrot in a food
   processor, if the mixture is a little dry add $^1/_3$ of the
   passata. Set aside.
2. In a large, deep non-stick fry pan, fry over a medium-
   high heat the onion and sausages until onion is
   transparent and sausages are slightly brown.
3. Add garlic and cubed vegetables, fry over a medium-
   high heat, turning occasionally for 5-10 minutes.
4. Add balance of ingredients and stir well.
5. Bring to boil, cover and simmer for 30 minutes or until
   potatoes are soft.

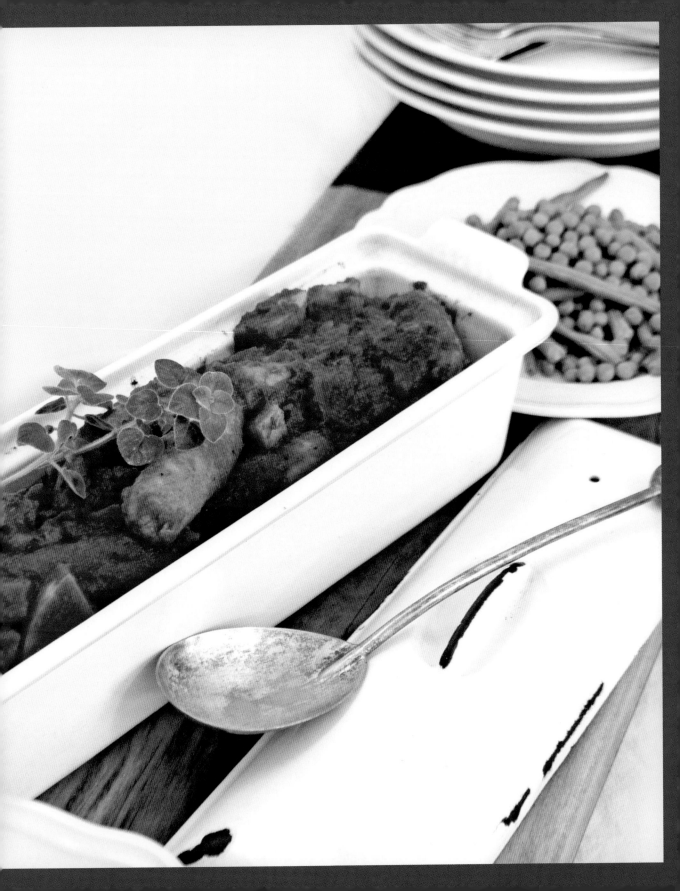

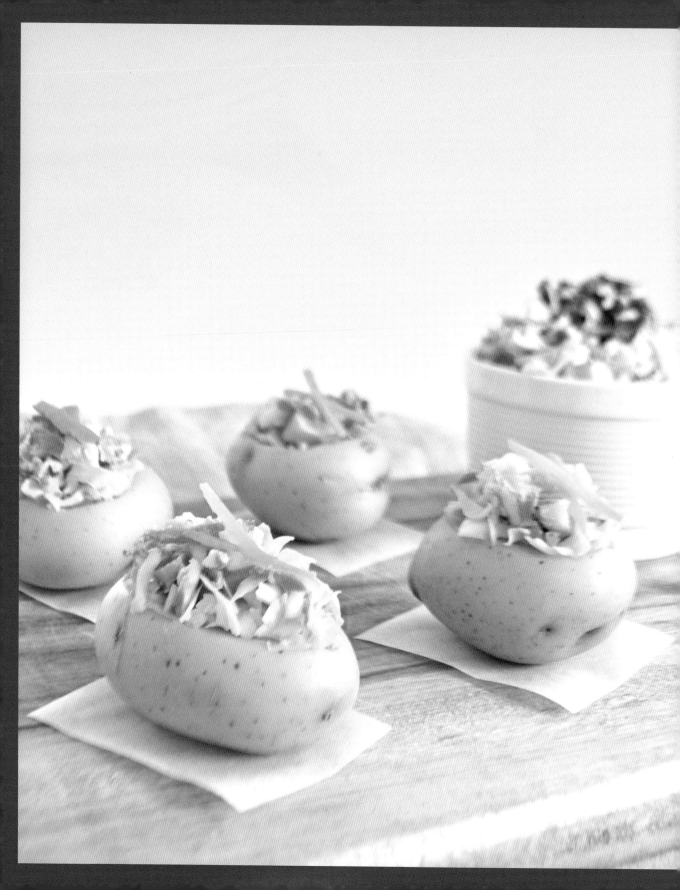

Potatoes and Waldorf Slaw

SERVES TWO ADULTS AND TWO CHILDREN FOR A LIGHT LUNCH, OR A GREAT SIDE FOR DINNER.
Scooped out potato can be used the following day in another dish.

4 small to medium-sized
  washed potatoes
180 g (7 oz) green cabbage,
  chopped finely
50 g (1.7 oz) raw walnuts,
  chopped roughly
½ green apple, diced small
2 heaped tablespoons
  Greek style yogurt

1. Boil potatoes whole until cooked through.
2. Remove from water with tongs and cut off top of potato and scoop out $\frac{1}{3}$ of the flesh. Set aside.
3. In a small mixing bowl combine balance of ingredients to make the slaw.
4. Spoon waldorf slaw into warm potatoes and serve.

Caesar Salad Soldiers

SERVES TWO TODDLERS OR ONE CHILD FOR A FUN LUNCH OR EASY DINNER

2 slices of wholemeal
   bread, cut into fingers
A small handful of
   parmesan or cheddar
   cheese
Vegetable spread (yeast
   extract) or similar
3 cherry tomatoes, cut in
   half
2 eggs
A few small cos lettuce
   leaves

1. Sprinkle cheese on the top half of each finger of bread and grill until cheese has melted.
2. Lay out fingers and spread vegetable spread on the bottom of each finger where there is no cheese. This will be the soldier's boots. With a toothpick add 2 eyes to the opposite end of each finger.
3. Place a cherry tomato half above the eyes as each soldier's helmet.
4. Place 2 eggs in a saucepan and cover with cold water, cover with lid.
5. Place on stove on a high heat and bring to the boil. Turn down to medium heat and simmer for 3 minutes exactly.
6. Remove eggs from water with a slotted spoon and place in egg cups. Slice the top off the eggs.
7. Arrange soldiers in a line and garnish with lettuce to create a field the soldiers are walking through.

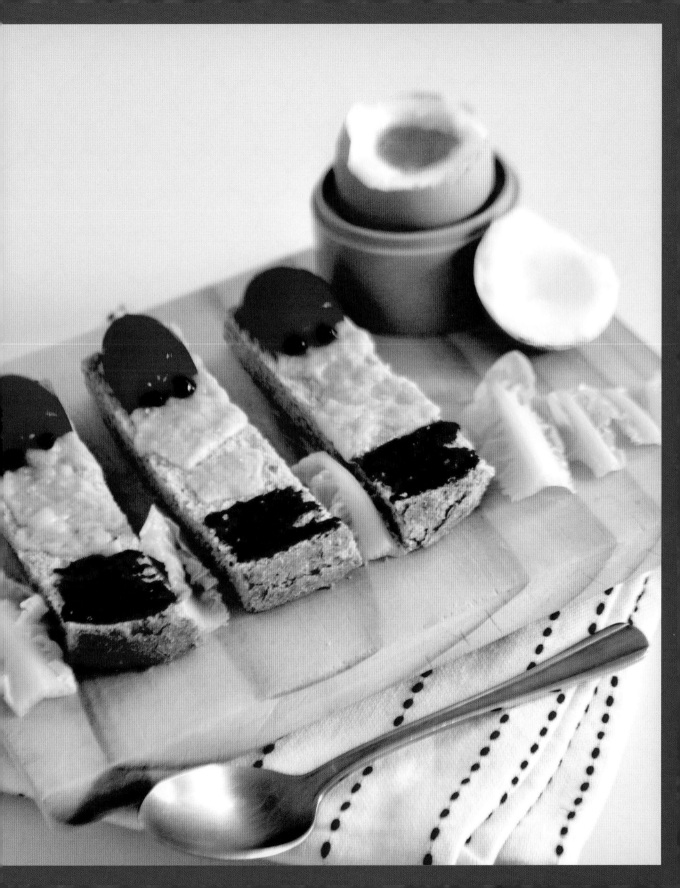

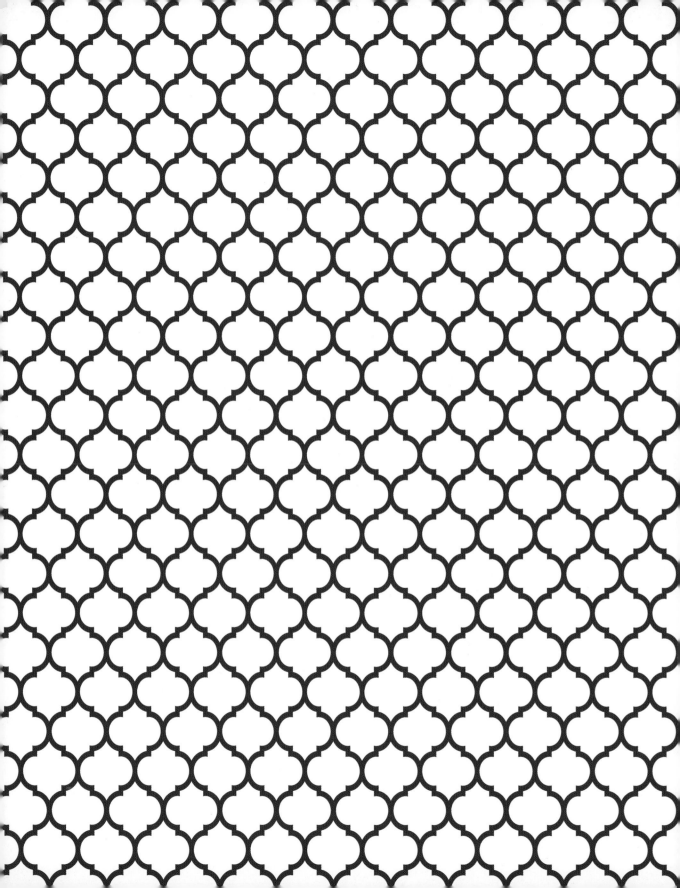

CHAPTER 5

Sweet Snacks

Sweets often seem to be the easiest snack option, but are sometimes the hardest to make healthy. This chapter has embraced our love for sweetness and harnessed the natural sugar and nutrients of fruit and vegetables to recreate our old favorites into healthier options that children (and adults) still enjoy.

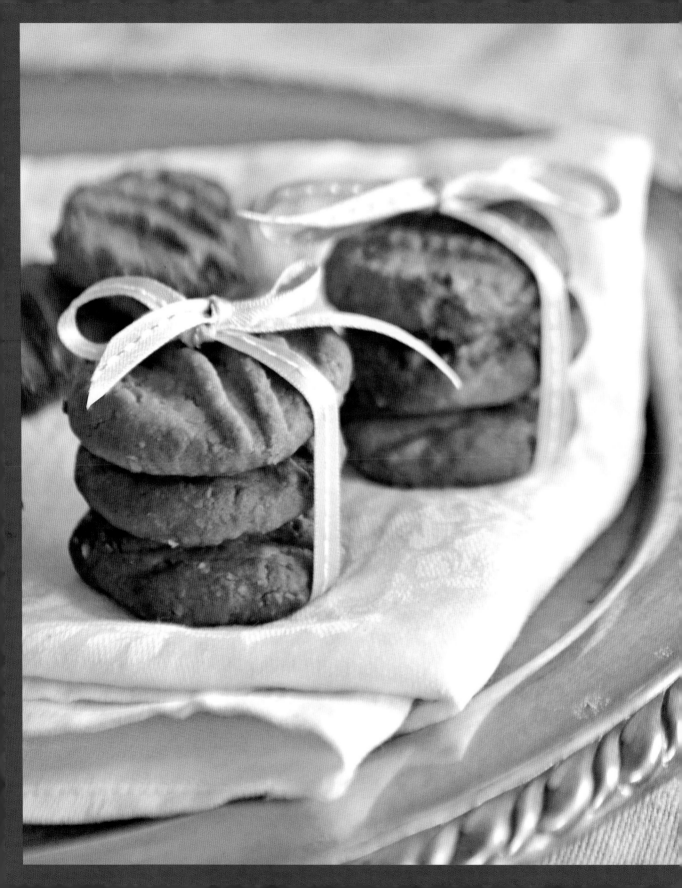

Peanut Butter and Honey Cookies

This recipe is quick and easy when unexpected guests arrive. Whilst it is free from added fats and refined sugars, it is still a 'sometimes' treat as it does have a generous amount of natural fat and sugar, but without the 'nasties' that store-bought biscuits have.

90 g (3 oz) peanut butter (100% peanuts)
2 dessertspoons honey
2 tablespoons boiling water
40 g (1½ oz) wholemeal self-raising flour

1. Preheat oven to 180°C/160°C fan forced (350°F/gas 4) and line 2 large baking trays with baking paper.
2. In a small mixing bowl combine all the wet ingredients well.
3. Add flour and mix through thoroughly.
4. Spoon out mixture with a teaspoon onto baking tray and gently push down each biscuit with a fork to flatten slightly. If the fork sticks simply wet the form with water. Bake for 10–15 minutes, or until golden brown.
5. Once slightly cooled, transfer onto a rack to cool completely.

Coconut Haystacks

MAKES 16 BITE-SIZE TREATS
A quick snack for a sweet tooth. This recipe is gluten, dairy and nut free.

1 heaped teaspoon honey
2 tablespoons coconut milk
50 g (1¾ oz) organic
  shredded coconut
1 egg white

1. Preheat oven to 150°C/130°C fan forced (300°F/gas 2) and line a large baking tray with baking paper.
2. Mix honey and coconut milk well in a small mixing bowl.
3. Add shredded coconut and combine gently ensuring all of the coconut is coated with the coconut milk mixture. Set aside.
4. In a separate mixing bowl beat egg white until soft peaks form. This can be done with a whisk, beaters or a fork.
5. Gently add and fold the coconut mixture into the egg white.
6. Spoon out mixture with a teaspoon onto baking tray. Bake for 20–25 minutes, or until golden brown.
7. Cool on baking tray.

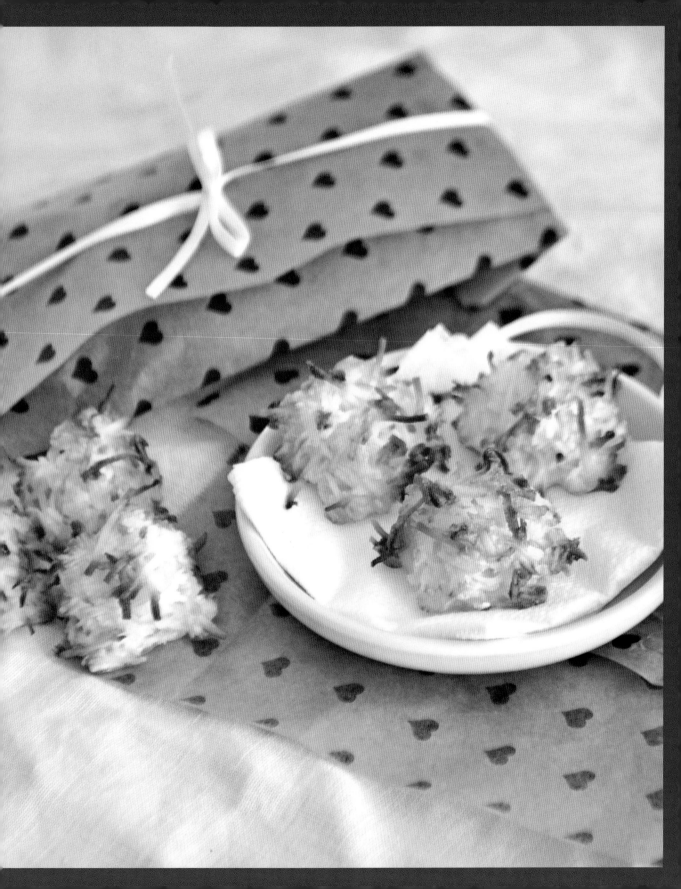

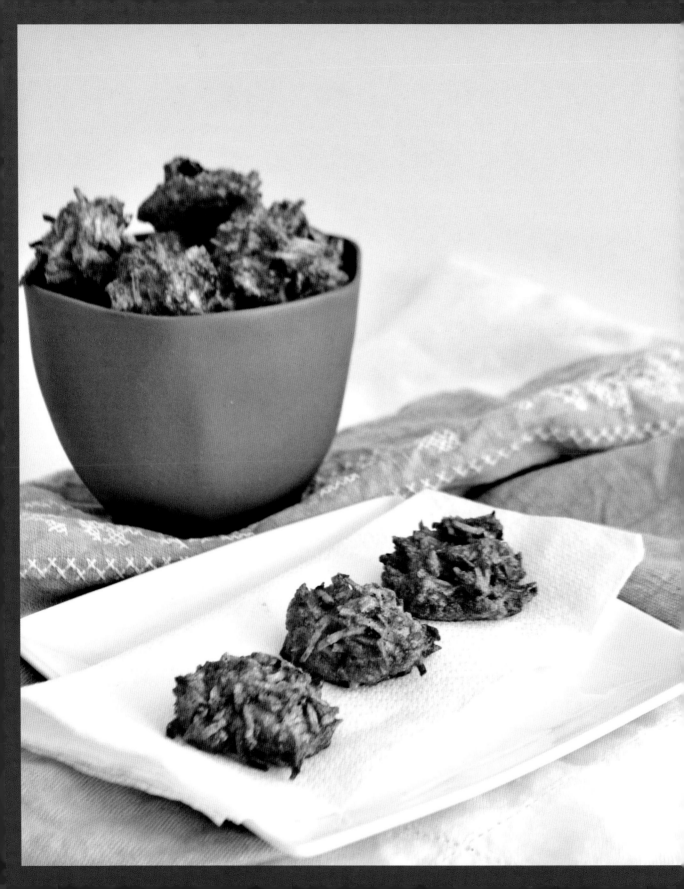

Coconut, Vanilla and Prune Macaroons

MAKES 12 BITE-SIZE TREATS

Great when unexpected guests arrive or for lunchboxes treats. This snack is gluten, dairy and nut free.

2 pitted and hydrated prunes (soak in a cup of water overnight in refrigerator or for 30 minutes in a cup of boiling water)

$\frac{1}{3}$ teaspoon vanilla bean paste

30 g (1 oz) organic shredded coconut

1 egg white

1. Preheat oven to 150°C/130°C fan forced (300°F/gas 2) and line a large baking tray with baking paper.
2. Dice hydrated prunes finely and place in a small mixing bowl.
3. Thoroughly combine with vanilla bean paste and shredded coconut. Set aside.
4. In a separate mixing bowl beat egg white until soft peaks form. This can be done with a whisk, beaters or a fork.
5. Gently add and fold the coconut mixture into the egg white.
6. Spoon out mixture with a teaspoon onto baking tray. Bake for 20–25 minutes, or until golden brown.
7. Cool on baking tray.

Nutty Bars

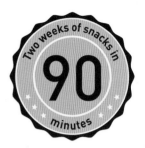

MAKES 10-12 BARS
Store in an airtight container.
Sesame seeds, pepitas (pumpkin seeds) or dried cranberries can be added
for variety.

90 g (3 oz) rolled oats
200 g (6½ oz) mixed nuts,
   chopped roughly
40 g (1½ oz) cornflakes
60 ml (2 fl oz) boiling water
2 tablespoons honey (if you
   have a sweet tooth you
   can double the amount of
   honey)
1 large egg white, whisked
   lightly

1. Preheat oven to 180°C/160°C fan forced (350°F/gas 4)
   and line a 20 x 20 x 5 cm (8 x 8 x 2 in) baking tin with
   baking paper.
2. Place oats and nuts in a non-stick frypan and stir over a
   medium heat until nuts and oats begin to roast slightly.
   These can also be roasted lightly in the oven.
3. Place nuts and oats in a large mixing bowl and add
   cornflakes, combine well. Set aside.
4. In a small bowl or jug mix boiling water and half of the
   honey until honey has dissolved into the water.
5. Add honey mixture to dry ingredients and mix
   thoroughly.
6. Add whisked egg white and mix through quickly.
7. Pour mixture into baking tin and spread out evenly.
   Push mixture down hard with a spatula or clean hands
   to ensure the mixture is dense and firm. Drizzle with
   balance of honey.
8. Bake for 20–30 minutes, or until firm and golden brown.
9. Cool completely and cut into fingers.

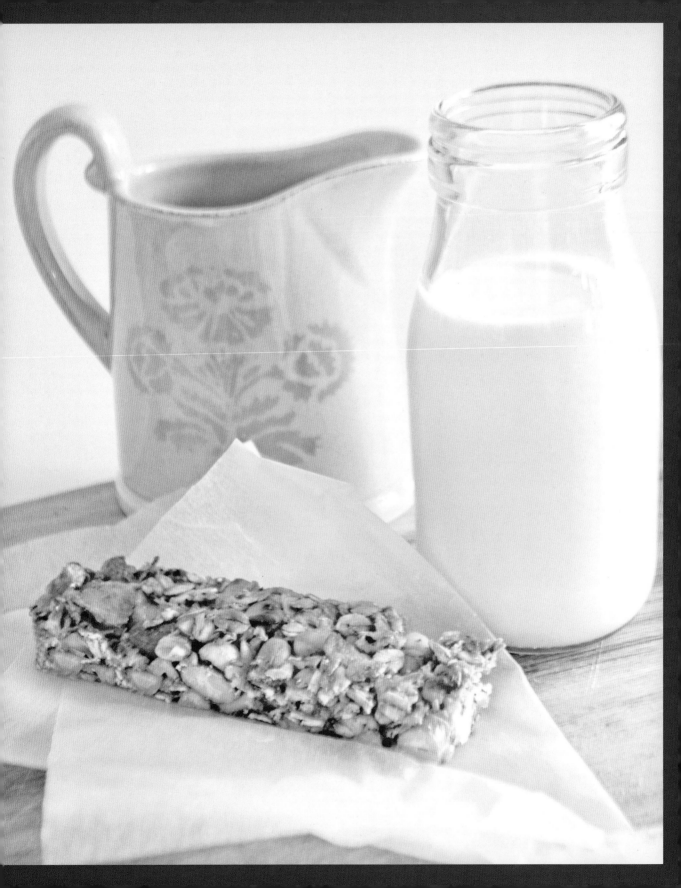

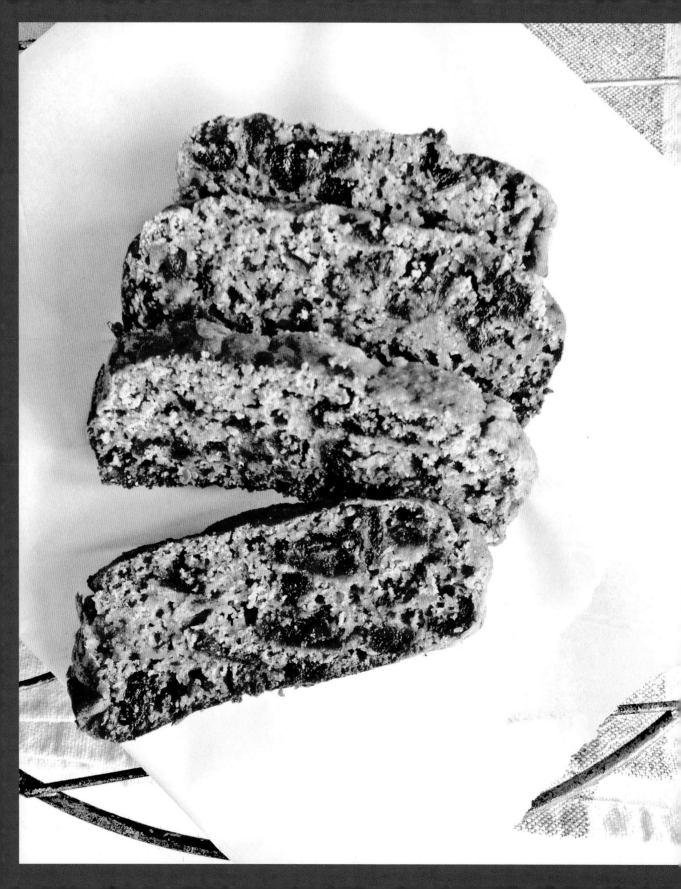

Friendly Date Cake

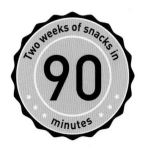

MAKES 10-12 SLICES

This is quite a moist, dense cake that can be stored in an airtight container for a couple of days or cut into fingers and frozen for lunchbox snacks.

135 g (4 ½ oz) rolled oats, blended into a fine flour

2 teaspoons baking powder

200 g (7 oz) chopped pitted dates (can mix with organic sultanas if desired)

3 heaped teaspoons of Greek style yogurt

125 ml (4 fl oz) milk

½ teaspoon vanilla bean extract

1. Preheat oven to 180°C/160°C fan forced (350°F/gas 4) and line a loaf tin with baking paper.
2. Mix dry ingredients and form a well in the mixture.
3. Add balance of ingredients, mix well and pour into baking tray.
4. Bake for 40–50 minutes. Press cake down and make sure it springs back up.
5. Remove from tin and put on a rack until cool.
6. Serve warm for a sweet dessert or cut into slices for a great morning tea snack.

Apple, Coconut and Oat Slice

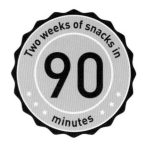

Two weeks of snacks in
90
minutes

MAKES 12 SLICES

This slice is slightly chewy on top and soft on the bottom – a perfect introduction to muesli bars for toddlers. Apple can be substituted with a small mashed banana or mashed pear for variety.

50 g (1½ oz) wholemeal self-raising flour
½ teaspoon baking powder
40 g (1½ oz) organic sultanas
70 g (2⅓ oz) rolled oats
30 g (1 oz) organic shredded coconut
½ teaspoon ground cinnamon
1 egg, whisked lightly
125 ml (4 fl oz) milk
1 red apple peeled and grated (use a zester grater)
1 dessertspoon honey

1. Preheat oven to 180°C/160°C fan forced (350°F/gas 4) and line a 20 x 20 x 5 cm (8 x 8 x 2 in) baking tin with baking paper.
2. In a mixing bowl combine all dry ingredients well.
3. Add egg, milk, grated apple and honey and mix through thoroughly.
4. Pour mixture into baking tin and spread out evenly. Bake for 25–30 minutes, or until golden brown.
5. Cut into fingers and serve.

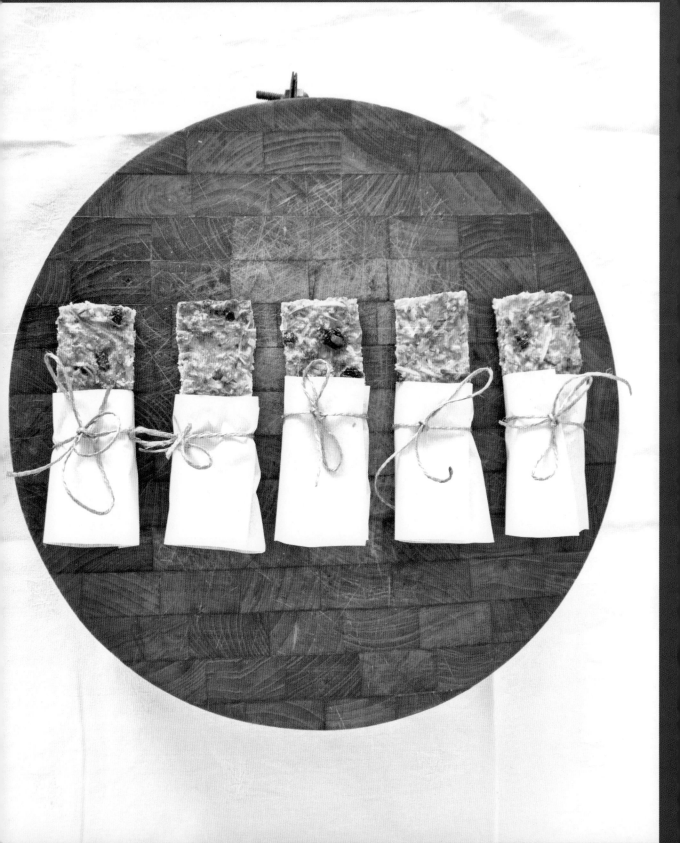

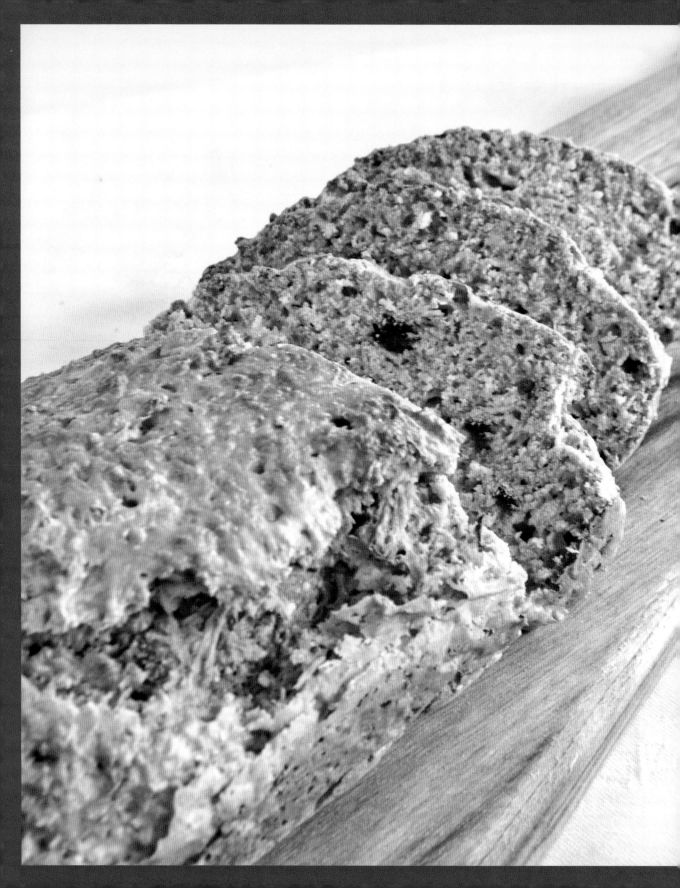

Fruity Bread

MAKES 10–12 SERVES

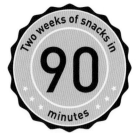

3 tablespoons organic sultanas

1 medium ripe banana, mashed

1 red apple, peeled and grated (use a zester grater)

⅓ zucchini (courgette), grated (use a zester grater)

225 g (7 ¼ oz) wholemeal self-raising flour

2 eggs, whisked lightly

1 dessertspoon honey

1 teaspoon ground cinnamon

1. Preheat oven to 180°C/160°C fan forced (350°F/gas 4) and line a loaf tin with baking paper.
2. Combine all ingredients in a large mixing bowl, mixing well. Pour into tin and bake for 30–40 minutes.
3. Remove from tin and put on a rack until cool.
4. Cut into slices and serve. (If younger children are finding it tricky to chew slightly firmer foods you can slice the top and/or sides off the loaf. I also like to place in layers with baking paper between the slices and freeze in a container.)
5. This bread can also be toasted with cream cheese or pear and raspberry jam.

Pancakes

MAKES 12-18 PANCAKES

Serves a family of four for breakfast, or can be made into smaller pikelets and frozen for lunchbox snacks.

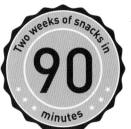

2 eggs

250 ml (8 fl oz) milk

75 g (2½ oz) pear, peeled and mashed or grated (use a zester grater)

1 red apple peeled, cored and grated (use a zester grater)

300 g (9½ oz) wholemeal self-raising flour

1 teaspoon butter

1. In a large mixing bowl whisk eggs well, add in milk, pear and apple. Mix until thoroughly combined.
2. Add flour and mix until there are no lumps.
3. Melt butter in non-stick frying pan on a medium heat. Ladle in first pancake. Once bubbles form around sides flip pancake and cook other side until golden.
4. Continue to cook pancakes with the remaining mixture.
5. Serve with cream and strawberries.

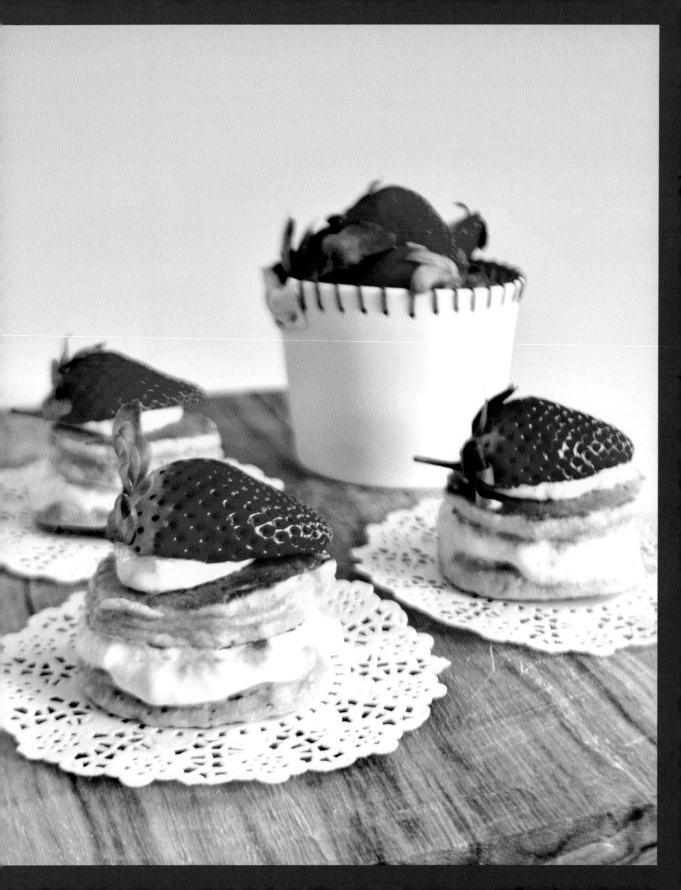

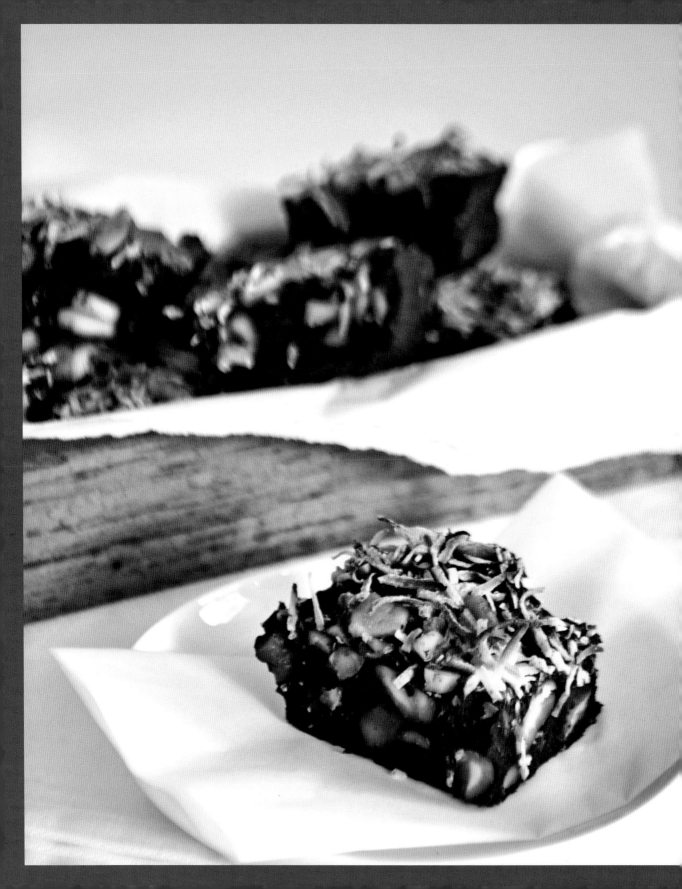

Cashew and Beetroot Brownies

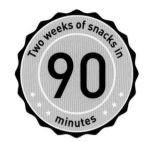

Two weeks of snacks in **90** minutes

MAKES 10 BROWNIES

Delicious served warm, and also great served at room temperature for lunchboxes. These brownies can also be frozen and thawed for school lunchbox treats.

Other nuts can be used if preferred.

20 g (¾ oz) raw peeled baby beetroot, grated

90 g (2 oz) (approx. 10) pitted prunes

80 ml (2 fl oz) coconut milk

2 dessertspoons honey (this can be doubled if you have a sweet tooth)

1 egg

50 g (1½ oz) wholemeal self-raising flour

20 g (¾ oz) cacao or cocoa powder

80 g (2¾ oz) cashew nuts, chopped roughly

Extra cashews chopped roughly, to sprinkle on top

2 heaped tablespoons organic shredded coconut, to sprinkle on top

1. Preheat oven to 180°C/160°C fan forced (350°F/gas 4) and line a loaf tin with baking paper.
2. Place beetroot, prunes, coconut milk, honey and egg in a food processor and blend until smooth.
3. Place flour, cocoa and cashew nuts in a mixing bowl, mix well.
4. Add pureed wet ingredients and combine.
5. Pour into loaf tin, sprinkle cashews and coconut on top and lightly press down into top of brownie mixture.
6. Bake for 20–30 minutes, until brownie mixture is firm to touch.

Tangy Apple Chips and Cinnamon Yogurt

SERVES TWO TODDLERS OR ONE CHILD

1 red apple
Juice of ½ a lime
90 g (3 oz) Greek style
  yogurt
1 teaspoon honey
Sprinkle of ground
  cinnamon

1. Peel and core apple, and cut into 'french fries' sticks.
2. Place in a bowl and pour lime juice over and mix through to ensure all apple chips are covered well.
3. In a separate small bowl place yogurt with honey and cinnamon on top. Swirl in honey and cinnamon with a toothpick.
4. Serve apple chips in a separate small ramekin and yogurt beside for dipping.

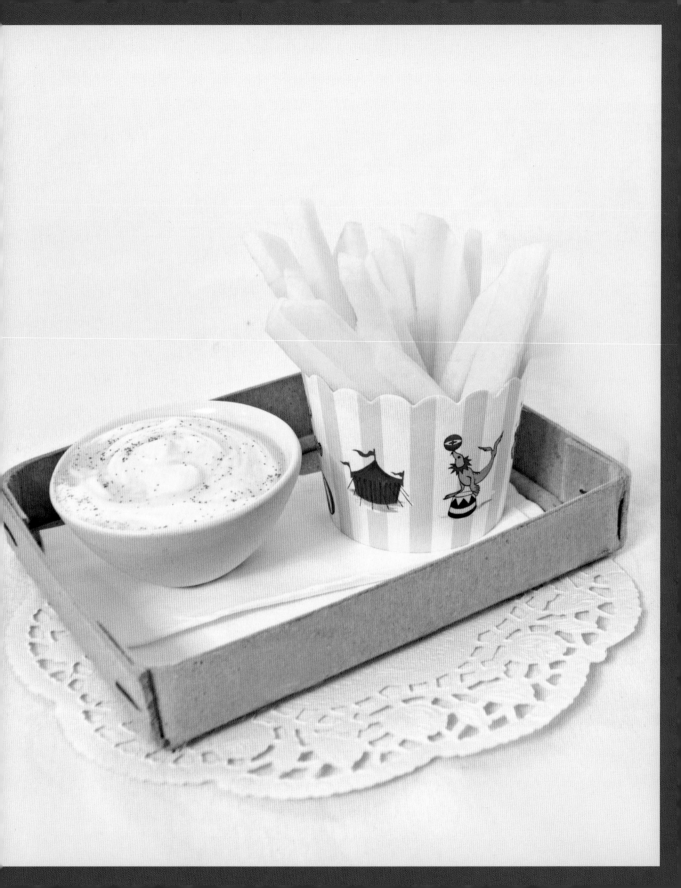

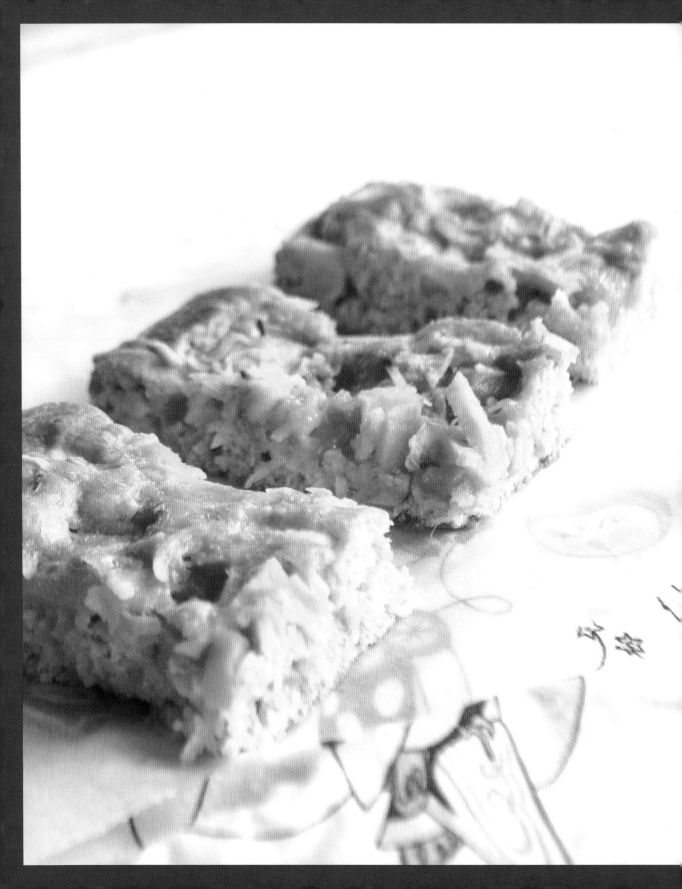

Apple and Mango Slice

MAKES 10-12 SERVES

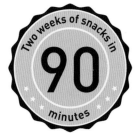

3 eggs
60 ml (2 fl oz) honey
70 g (2¼ oz) Greek style
  yogurt
125 ml (4 fl oz) milk
300 g (9½ oz) wholemeal
  self-raising flour
45 g (1½ oz) organic
  shredded coconut
2 apples, peeled, cored and
  chopped finely
1 mango, peeled and flesh
  chopped finely

1. Preheat oven to 180°C/160°C fan forced (350°F/gas 4) and line a 30 x 20 x 3.5 (13 x 10 x 2 in) baking tin with baking paper.
2. Whisk eggs in a large mixing bowl and add honey, yogurt and milk, mix well.
3. Add flour and two thirds of the coconut, mix well and pour into baking tray.
4. Combine chopped apples, mango and remaining coconut in a small bowl and spread over top of cake mixture, pressing down whilst spreading.
5. Bake for 25–35 minutes. Press cake down and make sure it springs back up.
6. Remove from tin and put on a rack until cool.
7. Cut into squares and freeze for easy snacks on the go or in lunchboxes.

Apple Juice and Almond Bites

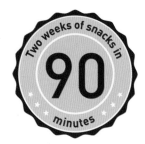

MAKES 20–24 BITE SIZE TREATS

These snacks are sweet little spongy snacks, great for car trips without the crumbs!

40 g (1½ oz) wholemeal self-raising flour

50 g (1¾ oz) rolled oats

125 ml (4 fl oz) 100% apple juice

½ small zucchini (courgette) (70 g (2⅓ oz)) finely grated (use a zester grater)

1 teaspoon honey

3 dessertspoons flaked almonds

extra flaked almonds, to decorate

1. Preheat oven to 180°C/160°C fan forced (350°F/gas 4) and line a large baking tray with baking paper.
2. In a mixing bowl thoroughly combine all ingredients except for almonds.
3. Fold almonds through mixture carefully.
4. Spoon out mixture with a teaspoon onto baking tray and gently push down to flatten slightly. Place 2–3 flaked almonds on top of each spoonful. Bake for 20–30 minutes, or until brown.
5. Transfer onto a cooling rack and store in an airtight container for a couple of days, or freeze.

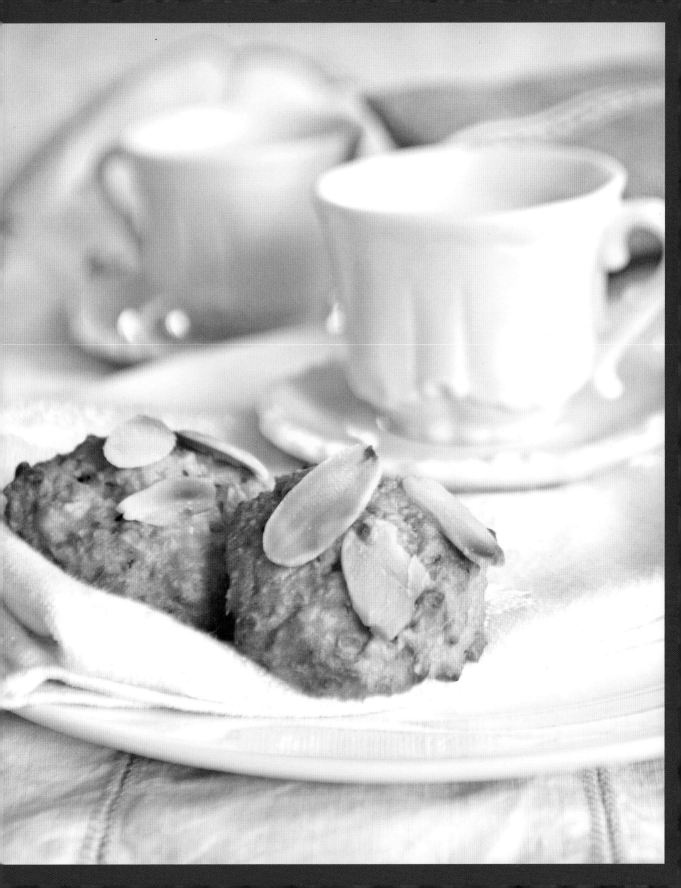

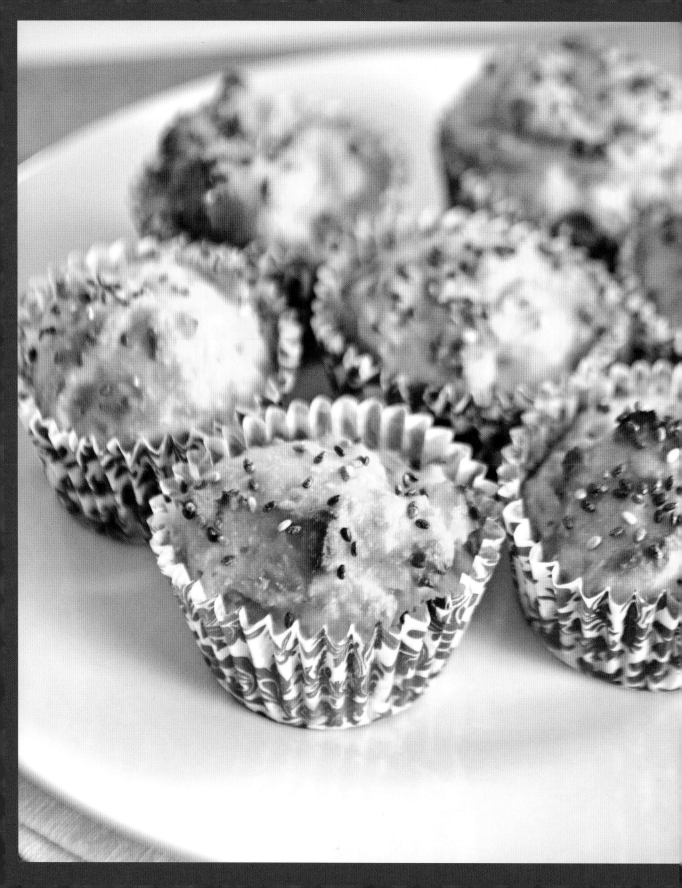

Carrot, Orange and Chia Seed Muffins

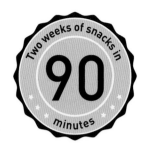

MAKES 10–12 MINI MUFFINS DEPENDING ON SIZE OF MUFFIN TRAY

Serve warm for an easy morning or afternoon tea snack, or store in an airtight container in the pantry or freezer for lunchbox snacks.

1 small carrot (approx. 70 g (2⅓ oz) finely grated (use zester grater))

Zest of a small orange

Juice of a small orange (90 ml (3 fl oz))

2 eggs

1 tablespoons honey

150 g (4¾ oz) wholemeal self-raising flour

½ teaspoon black chia or poppy seeds

Extra black chia or poppy seeds to decorate

1. Preheat oven to 180°C/160°C fan forced (350°F/gas 4) and line a mini muffin tray with muffin papers.
2. In a large mixing bowl mix all ingredients until combined, do not over-mix.
3. Spoon out mixture with a teaspoon into muffin tray and sprinkle with extra seeds.
4. Bake for 15–20 minutes, or until golden brown.

The 'Yes It's Good for You' Chocolate Pudding

MAKES 4 SMALL PUDDINGS

Perfect for an afternoon tea snack or dessert. Cow's milk can be substituted with almond or soy if preferred.

13 g (just under ½ oz) cornflour (cornstarch)
1 dessertspoon cacao or cocoa powder
60 ml (2 fl oz) water
60 ml (2 fl oz) coconut milk
180 ml (6 fl oz) milk
1 dessertspoon honey

1. Mix dry ingredients in a small saucepan and gradually add water to make a smooth paste.
2. Gradually whisk in coconut milk and full cream milk until well combined.
3. Turn small hotplate on high and whisk mixture continuously until thickened, add honey and continue to whisk for a couple of minutes whilst simmering.
4. Pour mixture into ramekins or jars and place lids on while hot.
5. Place in the fridge for at least a couple of hours until set.
6. Serve with diced banana and dried coconut.

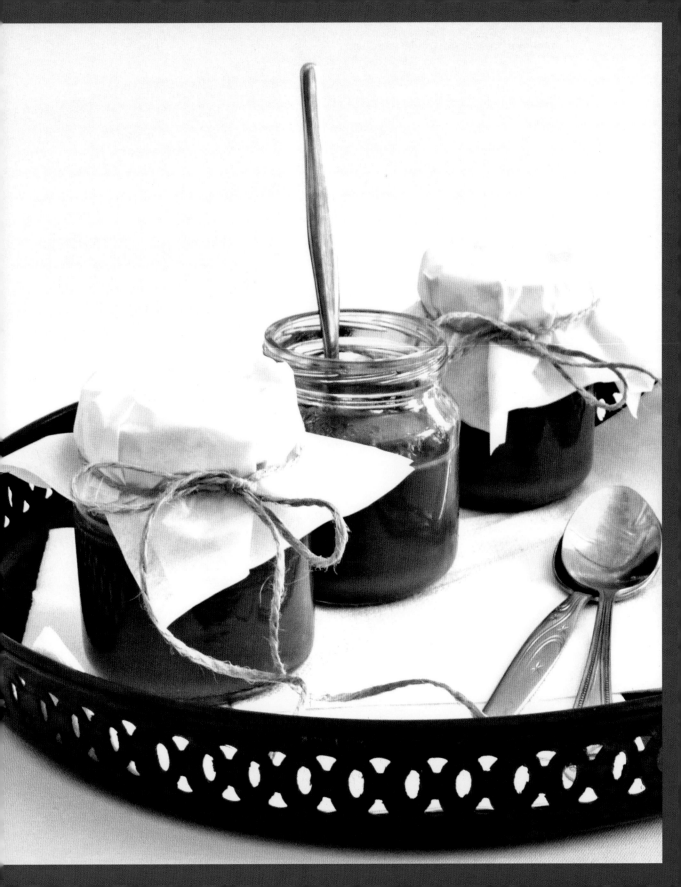

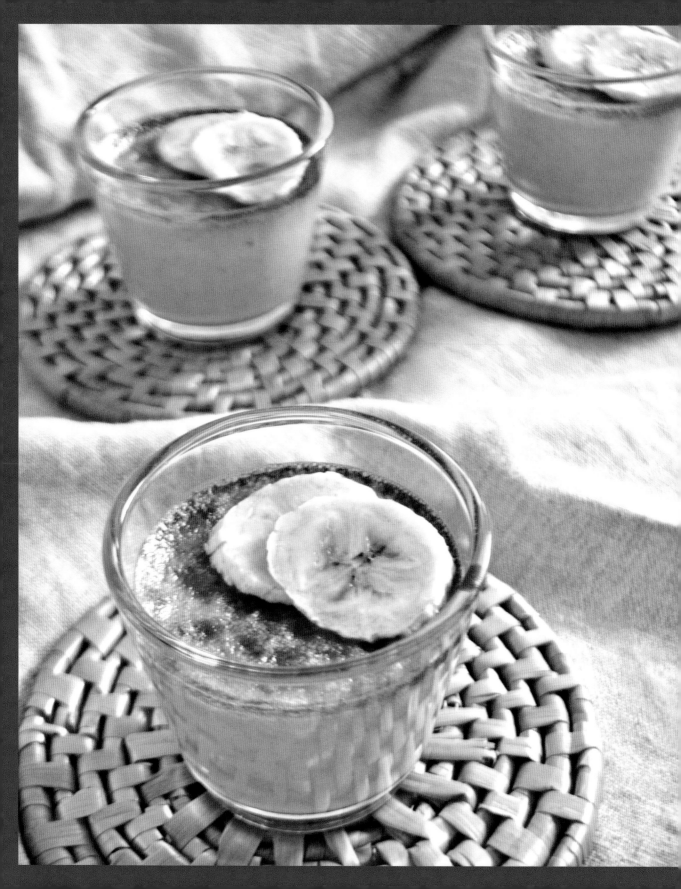

Baked Fruity Custard

MAKES 4–8 SERVES DEPENDING ON THE SIZE OF THE RAMEKIN USED

These custards can be eaten warm or cool. This snack will last in the fridge for a couple of days.

400 ml (13 fl oz) coconut milk
1 small apple peeled, cored
1 small ripe banana
4 eggs
2 teaspoon honey
2 teaspoon ground cinnamon

1. Preheat oven to 180°C/160°C fan forced (350°F/gas 4).
2. Place all ingredients in a blender and process until smooth.
3. Pour into small ramekins and place them in a baking tray half-filled with boiling water. Put in oven for 45 minutes.

Blueberry and Vanilla Treat

MAKES 4 SMALL PUDDINGS

Cow's milk can be substituted with coconut, almond or soy if preferred and other frozen berries can be used instead of blueberries if desired.

2 tablespoons cornflour (cornstarch)
250 ml (8 fl oz) milk
1 teaspoon vanilla bean paste
1 dessertspoon honey
20–30 frozen blueberries

1. Place cornflour in a small saucepan and gradually add milk to make a smooth paste.
2. Gradually whisk in balance of milk, vanilla bean paste and honey until well combined.
3. Turn small hotplate on high and whisk mixture continuously until thickened, continue to whisk for a couple of minutes whilst simmering.
4. Pour mixture into small ramekins or jars.
5. With the end of a teaspoon, push 5-6 blueberries into each pudding randomly.
6. Place in the fridge for at least a couple of hours until set.

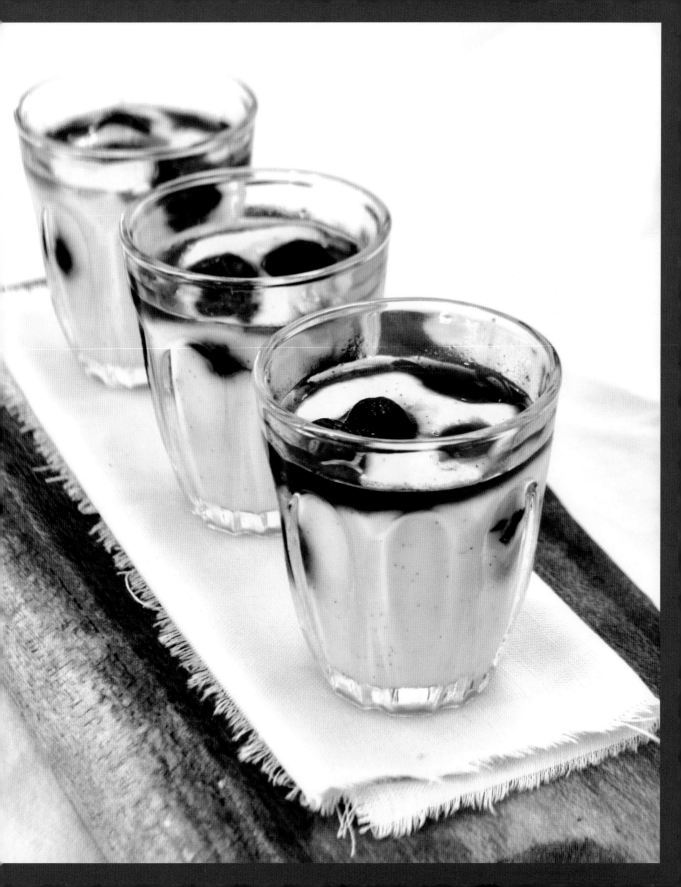

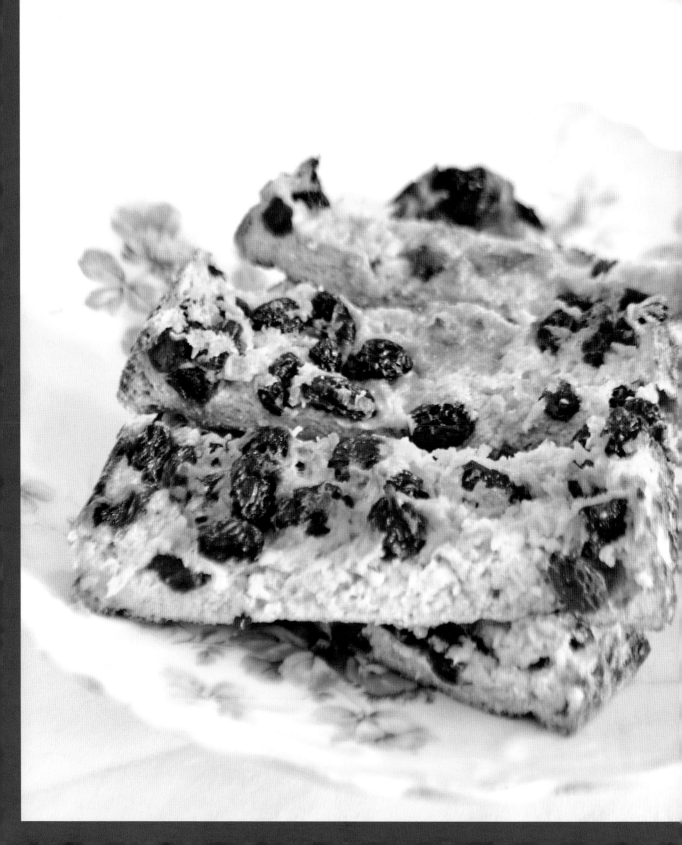

Bread and Apple Pudding

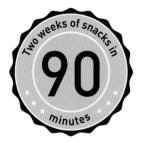

MAKES 10-12 SERVES

This snack can be eaten warm or cold, stored in the fridge for a couple of days or in the freezer for easy lunchbox treats.

50 g (1¾ oz) organic sultanas

125 ml (4 fl oz) boiling water

3 slices wholemeal bread (medium cut)

1 egg, whisked lightly

180 ml (6 fl oz) milk

1 red apple peeled, cored and grated (use a zester grater)

1. Place sultanas into a small ramekin and pour boiling water to cover, this will hydrate sultanas while you prepare the rest of the ingredients.
2. Preheat oven to 180°C/160°C fan forced (350°F/gas 4) and line a loaf tin with baking paper.
3. Cut crusts off bread and line the loaf tin with slices. (You may need to cut slices into wedges or in half to fill the dish evenly.)
4. In a small mixing bowl whisk egg, milk, grated apple and drained sultanas together.
5. Pour mixture over bread slices and gently massage into bread to ensure an even coverage. Bake for 40 minutes.
6. Cut into fingers and serve. (I like to place the slices in layers with baking paper between them and freeze in a container.)

Apple and Strawberry Jellies

MAKES 4

4 ripe strawberries
gelatine (preservative free
  is preferred)
boiling water
100 ml (3⅓ fl oz) 100%
  apple juice

1. Wash and remove tops from strawberries and place one in each of 4 small ramekins or glasses.
2. Place desired amount of gelatine in a small heat-proof measuring jug to make 125 ml (4 fl oz) of jelly in total. (Refer to instructions on gelatine packet.)
3. Pour approximately 20–30 ml (1 fl oz) of boiling water over the gelatine and whisk thoroughly until all the gelatine has dissolved.
4. Top up measuring jug with apple juice to make a total of 125 ml (4 fl oz) of jelly, whisk in well.
5. Pour over the strawberries into the ramekins or glasses and place in the refrigerator to set for at least a few hours, but preferably overnight.
6. Serve cold for a special treat or dessert.

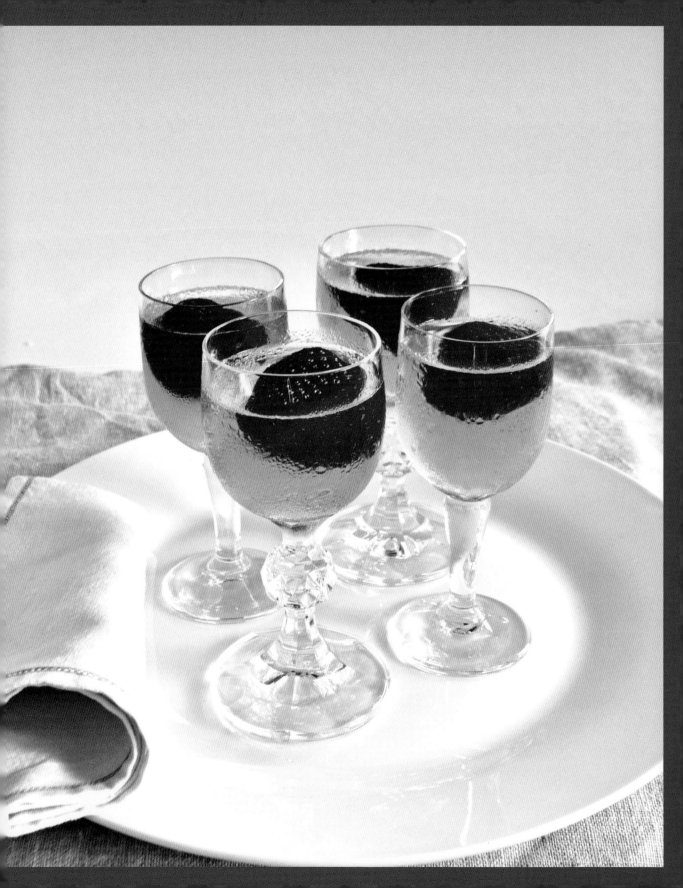

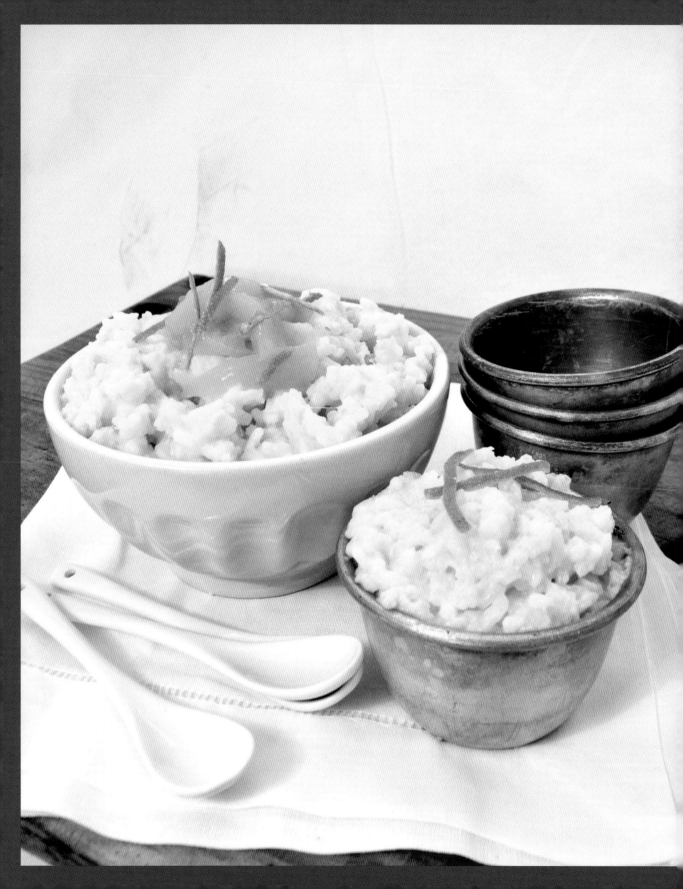

Coconut and Lime Rice Pudding

SERVES TWO ADULTS AND TWO CHILDREN, WITH COLD LEFTOVERS FOR MORNING OR AFTERNOON TEA THE FOLLOWING DAY FOR TWO CHILDREN.

If you have leftover rice from the night before this rice can be used, you will need 300–350 g (11 oz) of cooked rice.

90 g (3 oz) rice
250 ml (8 fl oz) coconut milk
440 g (15 oz) tinned mango cheeks or slices in natural juice
1 lime

1. In a medium saucepan boil rice until soft.
2. Drain rice but do not rinse.
3. Return pan to the stove and add coconut milk and can of mango juice and cheeks leaving one cheek aside for garnishing at the end.
4. Bring the rice mixture to the boil and simmer, stirring occasionally for approximately 15 minutes, or until the mixture has reduced and is thick and creamy.
5. Take off the heat and add the zest of the lime and a squeeze of lime juice. Stir well and serve.

Baked Apples

Because this dish requires a long baking time, it is a good idea to cook with other oven-baked meals such as a roast dinner. The cooking temperature can be lowered for this recipe, and cooking time simply extended to suit.

60 g (2 oz) chopped prunes
   or dates
water
4 medium sized red apples
60 g (2 oz) mixed nuts
   chopped roughly
30 g (11 oz) organic
   shredded coconut

1. Preheat oven to 200°C/180°C fan forced (400°F/gas 6) and line a 20 x 20 x 5 cm (8 x 8 x 2 in) baking tin with baking paper.
2. Place dates and/or prunes in a small saucepan and just cover with water. Bring to boil and simmer uncovered until soft and falling apart. Set aside.
3. Cut the top quarter of each apple off, peel the top portion and grate the flesh. Set grated flesh aside.
4. Core the apples well, only leaving 1 cm (½ in) thickness of apple as a baking cup for the stuffing.
5. In a small mixing bowl combine nuts, coconut, grated apple and prunes or dates including the infused cooking water.
6. Stuff apples with the mixture, mounding over the top of the cut apple. Place in baking tray and cover with foil, bake for at least 60 minutes, or until apple is soft.
7. Serve warm as a dessert or special occasion snack.

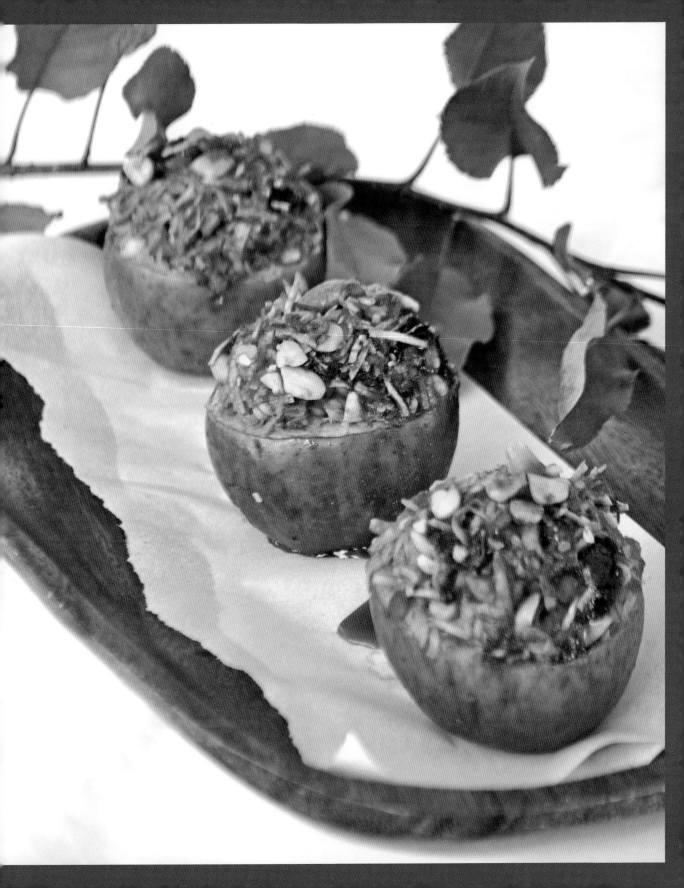

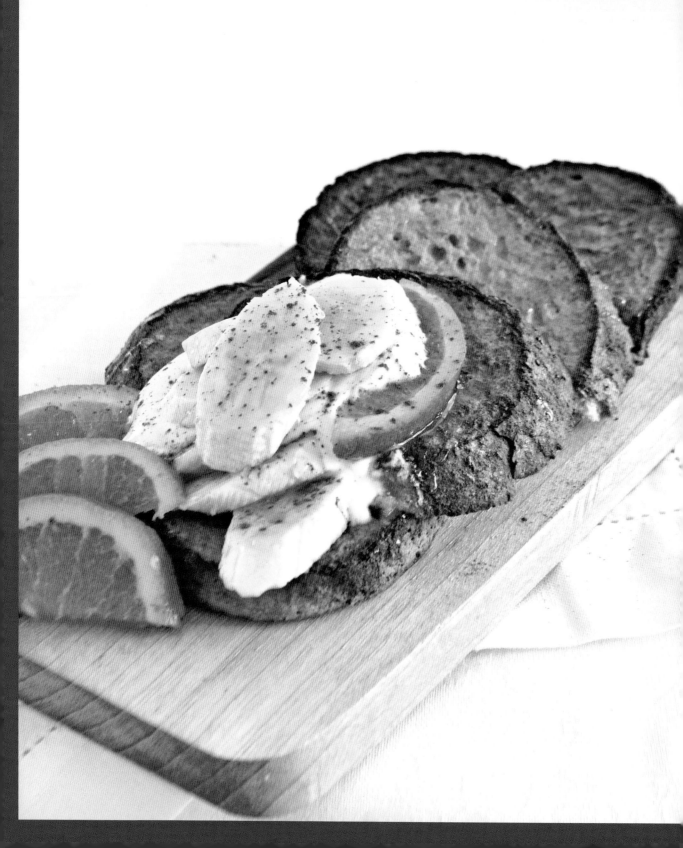

French Toast with a Twist

SERVES TWO ADULTS AND TWO CHILDREN FOR A TASTY AND NUTRITIOUS WEEKEND BREAKFAST,
OR AFTERNOON TEA SNACK.

1 ripe banana
125 g (4 oz) raw pumpkin
   peeled and seeded
2 eggs
½ teaspoon ground
   cinnamon
1 teaspoon honey
6 slices of wholemeal
   bread, thickly sliced
1 orange
Honey, Greek style yogurt,
   ground cinnamon and
   fresh fruit to serve

1. Preheat oven to 200°C/180°C fan forced (400°F/gas 6) and line 2 large baking trays with baking paper.
2. Puree banana and raw pumpkin in a food processor until smooth.
3. Add eggs, cinnamon and honey and process until well combined.
4. Pour egg mixture into a bowl and dip bread in it, soaking each slice well.
5. Place slices of soaked bread on lined baking trays separately and place in oven for 15-20 minutes or until golden brown.
6. Remove from oven and squeeze a light drizzle of orange juice over the toast.
7. Serve with honey, Greek style yogurt, cinnamon and fresh fruit.

Apple and Cinnamon Swirl Yogurt

SERVES TWO CHILDREN FOR A SWEET SNACK

1 apple peeled, cored and sliced thinly

Water

½ teaspoon ground cinnamon

6 tablespoons Greek style yogurt

1. Place apple slices in a small saucepan and cover with water.
2. Bring to boil and simmer until soft and water has evaporated – add extra water and continue cooking if apples are still firm once water has evaporated.
3. Transfer stewed apples into a small bowl and add cinnamon, mix well. Chill in refrigerator.
4. Place 3 tablespoons of yogurt in two separate dishes, spoon half of the apple mixture into each dish and swirl to mix.

Nectarine Yogurt with Coconut-Oat Crunch

SERVES TWO CHILDREN FOR A SNACK OR SPECIAL DESSERT

1 tablespoon quick oats

1 tablespoon organic shredded coconut

1 dessertspoon flaked almonds

1 teaspoon honey

1 ripe nectarine

6 tablespoons Greek style yogurt

1. Place oats, coconut and almonds in a small non-stick frypan and stir over a medium heat until golden brown.
2. Add honey and mix through thoroughly.
3. Pour mixture onto a sheet on non-stick paper and chill in the refrigerator.
4. Slice nectarine and arrange in two small bowls.
5. Add 3 tablespoons of yogurt into each bowl.
6. Top with crunchy oat mixture and serve.

Mixed Berry Yogurt

SERVES TWO CHILDREN FOR A QUICK AND HEALTHY MORNING OR AFTERNOON TEA SNACK

4 tablespoons of mixed berries (fresh or frozen)

6 tablespoons Greek style yogurt

1. In a small mixing bowl combine 2 tablespoons of berries and the yogurt.
2. Divide mixture into two small serving bowls and top with remaining berries.

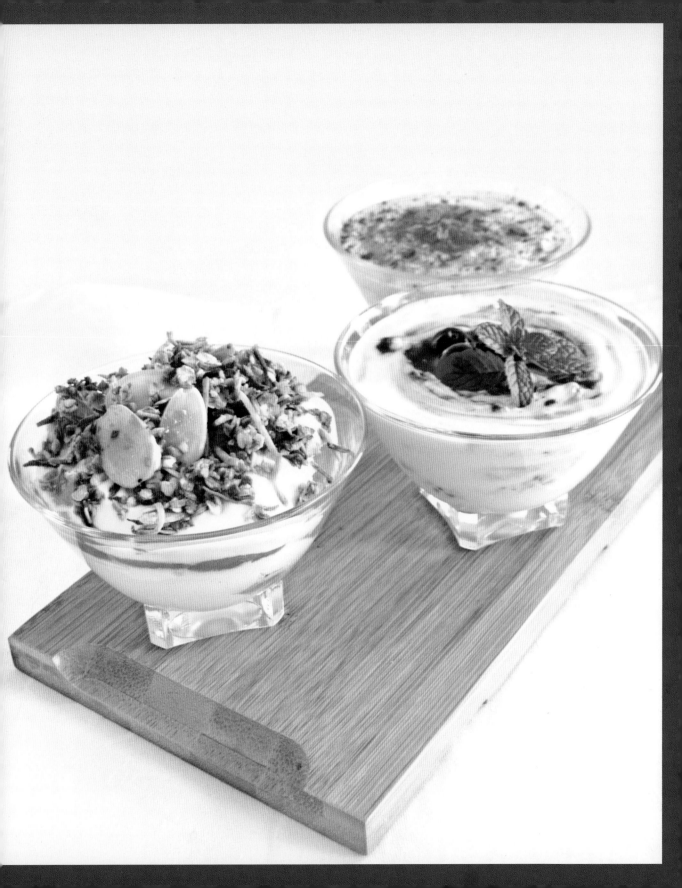

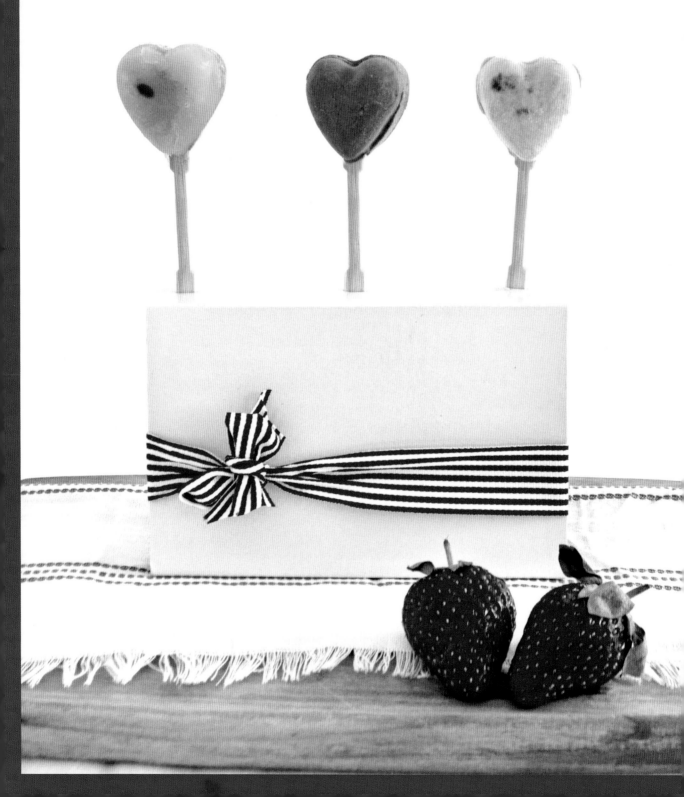

Icy Poles

Orange and Passionfruit Icy Poles

MAKES APPROXIMATELY 4–6 MINI-ICY POLES

1 large orange
1 passionfruit

1. Juice orange and mix well with pulp of passionfruit in a small bowl.
2. Spoon or pour into shaped silicone ice cube trays and place in freezer.
3. Check mixture after 15–20 minutes, once the mixture begins to harden insert paddle-pop sticks or rounded hors d'oeuvre sticks. Return to freezer until set.

Strawberry and Yogurt Icy Poles

MAKES APPROXIMATELY 4–6 MINI-ICY POLES

2 large ripe strawberries
2 tablespoons Greek style
  yogurt
2 teaspoons honey

1. Mash strawberries with a fork and mix well with yogurt and honey.
2. Spoon into shaped silicone ice cube trays and place in freezer.
3. Check mixture after 15–20 minutes, once the mixture begins to harden insert paddle-pop sticks or rounded hors d'oeuvre sticks. Return to freezer until set.

Chocolate and Coconut Icy Poles

MAKES APPROXIMATELY 8-10 MINI-ICY POLES

165 ml (5 ½ fl oz) light
  coconut milk
3 level teaspoons cacao or
  cocoa powder
5 teaspoons honey

1. Place all ingredients in a blender and mix until well combined.
2. Pour into shaped silicone ice cube trays and place in freezer.
3. Check mixture after 15–20 minutes, once the mixture begins to harden insert paddle-pop sticks or rounded hors d'oeuvre sticks. Return to freezer until set.

Watermelon Wands

This is a great snack for the children to help create. Other fruits such as grapes or fresh blueberries can also be used, cubed fruit can be used instead of melon balls.

2 large slices of seedless
   watermelon
½ honeydew melon
6 strawberries

1. Using a star shaped cookie cutter, cut 6 star shapes of watermelon on a chopping board. Set aside.
2. Using a melon baller, make 12 honeydew balls. Set aside.
3. Wash and cut the tops off the strawberries, set aside.
4. Using skewers or paper straws, slide fruit onto skewers or paper straws in desired order, and top with watermelon star.

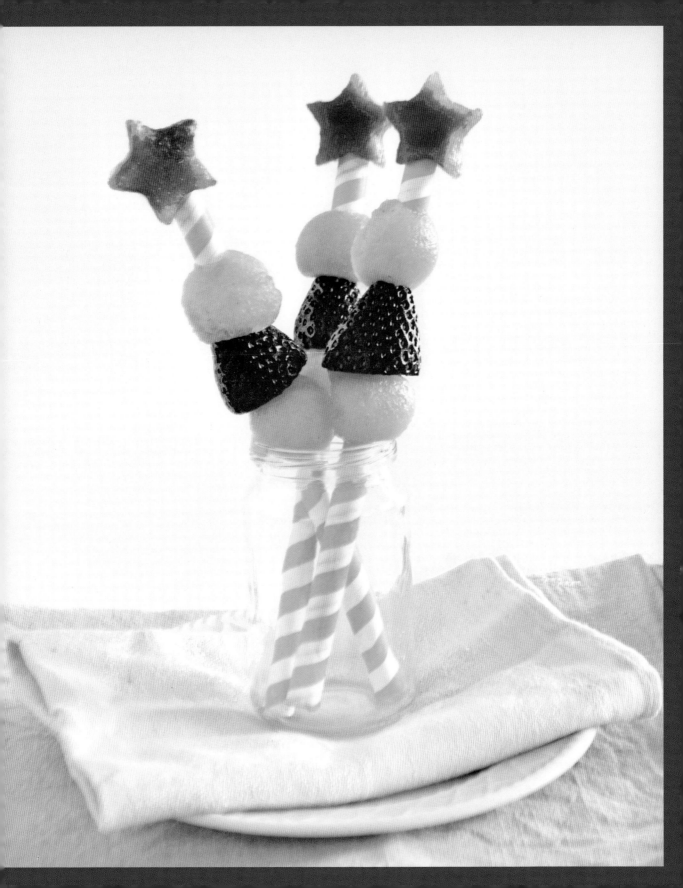

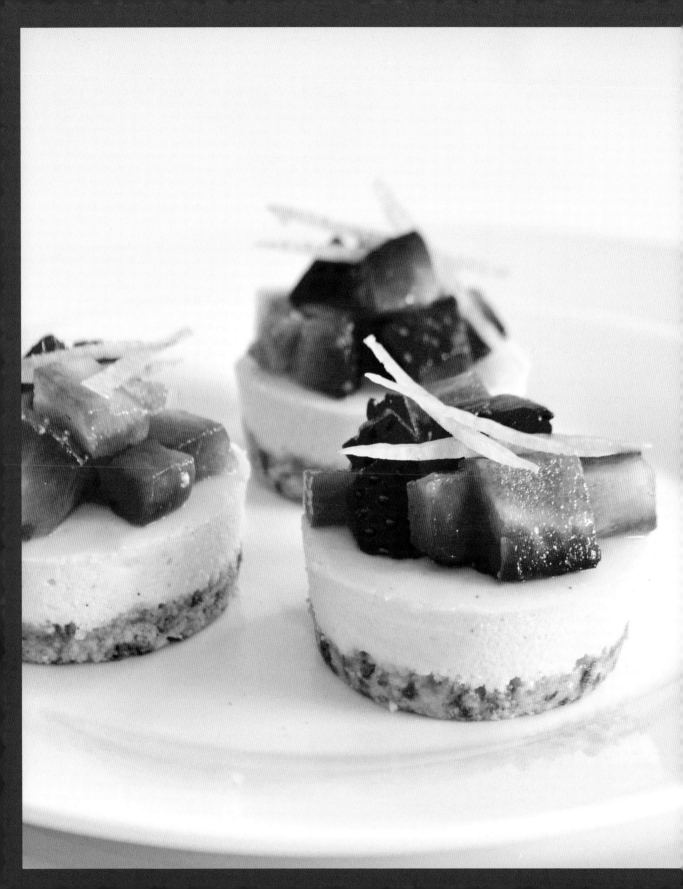

Lemon Cheesecakes

MAKES 12–20 DEPENDING ON SIZE OF MUFFIN TRAY USED.
This delicious cheesecake is gluten free and can be served as a special dessert or party treat. Whilst free from refined sugars and added fats, this sweet contains a large percentage of natural dairy fat, so the small serving portions of the mini-muffin trays are ideal. This can also be baked as a whole cheesecake in a pie tin.

Base
125 g (4 oz) unsalted
   cashew nuts
60 g (2 oz) dates

Cheesecake
250 g (8 oz) cream cheese
   (at room temperature)
80 g (2¾ oz) Greek style
   yogurt
60 ml (2 fl oz) honey
½ teaspoon vanilla bean
   extract
Zest of ½ lemon
1 tablespoon fresh lemon
   juice
1 egg
1 tablespoon cornflour
   (cornstarch)

Fresh strawberries to
   garnish

1. Preheat oven to 160°C/140°C fan forced (325°F/gas 3) and lightly spray a mini-muffin tray with olive oil. A silicone mini-muffin tray is also suitable for this recipe.
2. In a food processor, blend nuts and dates until they are well combined and the mixture starts sticking together.
3. Spoon out mixture into base of muffin tin and pack in firmly to make bases that are approximately ½ cm (¼ in) thick. Chill in refrigerator.
4. In a clean food processor, mix the cream cheese on a low setting until it becomes smooth.
5. Gradually add the balance of ingredients one at a time until well combined. Be sure to use a spatula to push the filling down from the sides of the food processor bowl, this will ensure a smooth and even consistency. Set aside.
6. Place bases in the oven and bake for 5–10 minutes, or until golden brown.
7. Remove from oven and spoon in cheesecake mixture.
8. Return to oven and bake for 20–30 minutes, until the cheesecake mixture has firmed enough to only have a slight wobble. Cooking time will depend on the size of the muffin tin.
9. Turn oven off and leave cheesecakes in oven until room temperature, then transfer into fridge.
10. Serve chilled with diced strawberries and lemon zest on top.

Merry Munchies

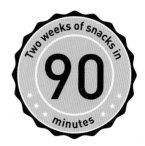

MAKES 10–12 SMALL BALLS

This is a great healthy treat for children and adults, a good idea for parties too.

40 g (1⅓ oz) organic
  sultanas
30 g (1 oz) organic shredded
  or desiccated coconut
30 g (1 oz) mixed nuts
  (cashews, almonds, brazil
  nuts etc)
4 pitted prunes
30 g (1 oz) rice bubbles/
  puffs
4 teaspoons water
Pinch ground cinnamon
Extra organic desiccated
  coconut for rolling balls in

1. In a small blender or food processor, process raisins, coconut, nuts, prunes and ⅓ of the rice bubbles until all ingredients are ground well.
2. Transfer this mixture into a bowl and combine with water and cinnamon.
3. Fold through remaining rice bubbles.
4. Using a heaped dessertspoon, form small balls and roll into coconut. Refrigerate until firm.

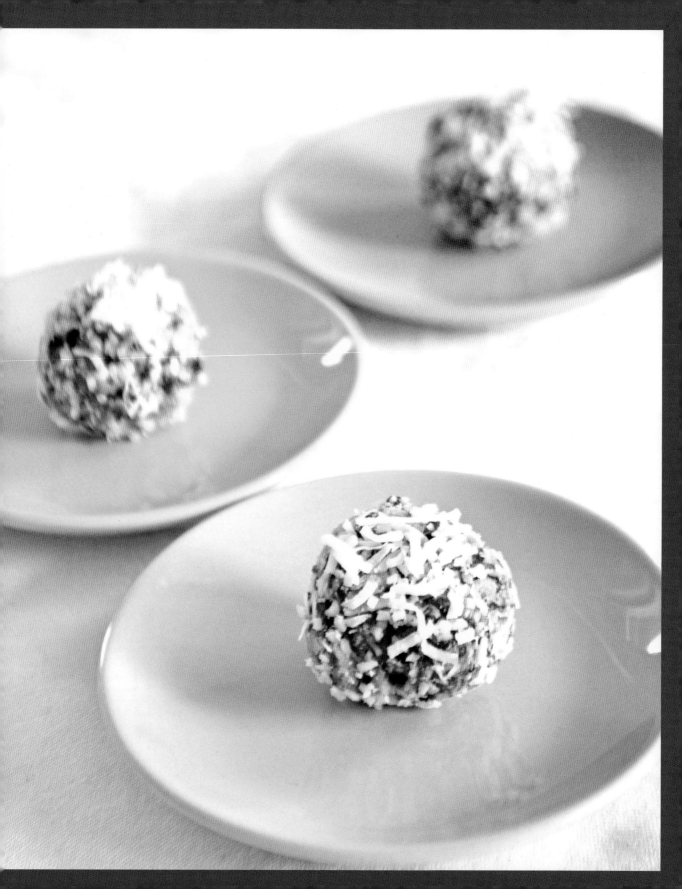

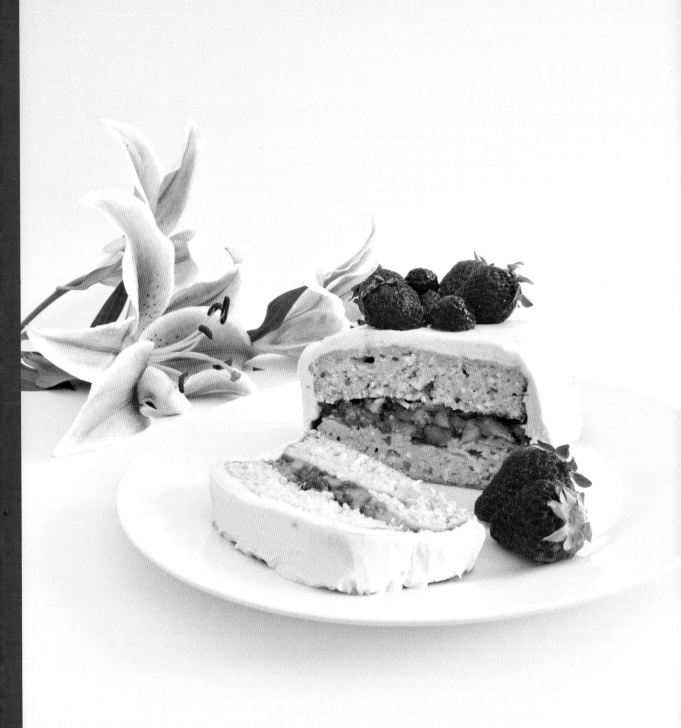

First Birthday Cake

SERVES 15-20
This is quite a dense and moist cake, best eaten fresh.

Cake

3 red apples peeled, cored and grated (use a zester grater)
4 tablespoons honey
15 g (½ oz) shredded coconut
190 g (6 ¼ oz) wholemeal self-raising flour
3 eggs
Fresh fruit to decorate

Filling

400 g (13 oz) canned pear halves in natural juice (no added sugar)
45 g (1 ½ oz) frozen raspberries

Icing

45 g (1 ½ oz) frozen raspberries (to tint the icing pink but you can substitute with other natural colors)
500 g (1 lb) cream cheese
125 ml (4 fl oz) honey

The night before the birthday, prepare:

Filling

1. Drain pear halves and chop into small pieces or mash lightly with a fork. Mash through frozen raspberries. Store in fridge overnight.

Icing

1. Sieve raspberries through a fine strainer to remove seeds, set aside.
2. Place cream cheese in a food processor, mix until smooth. Gradually add honey to taste and the raspberry or other colored ingredient. Store in fridge overnight.

On the birthday morning:

1. Preheat oven to 180°C/160°C fan forced (350°F/gas 4) and line 2 loaf tins with baking paper.
2. Place grated apples and honey in a small saucepan. Stir over low heat to melt honey and mix with apples. Set aside.
3. Separate eggs and beat whites until soft peaks form.
4. Mix coconut and flour in a mixing bowl, pour in honey and apple mixture, mix.
5. Add egg yolks, mix, then fold through beaten egg whites.
6. Pour into tins and bake for 25–35 minutes. Press cake down and make sure it springs back up.
7. Remove from tin and put on a rack until cool.
8. Cut one cake as per diagram (opposite page) to make a number '1'.
9. Cut all cakes in half and fill with prepared pear and raspberry filling.
10. Join and ice cake. Decorate as you wish.
11. Sing Happy Birthday to your special little one year old!

CHAPTER 6

Smoothies, Hot Drinks and Shakes

Refreshing smoothies, shakes and warming hot drinks feature in this chapter. Healthy drinks are an excellent way of increasing our intake of nutrients each day. Smoothies and shakes can be stored in reusable squeeze pouches for younger children and even taken to daycare or school for a snack if refrigeration is available.

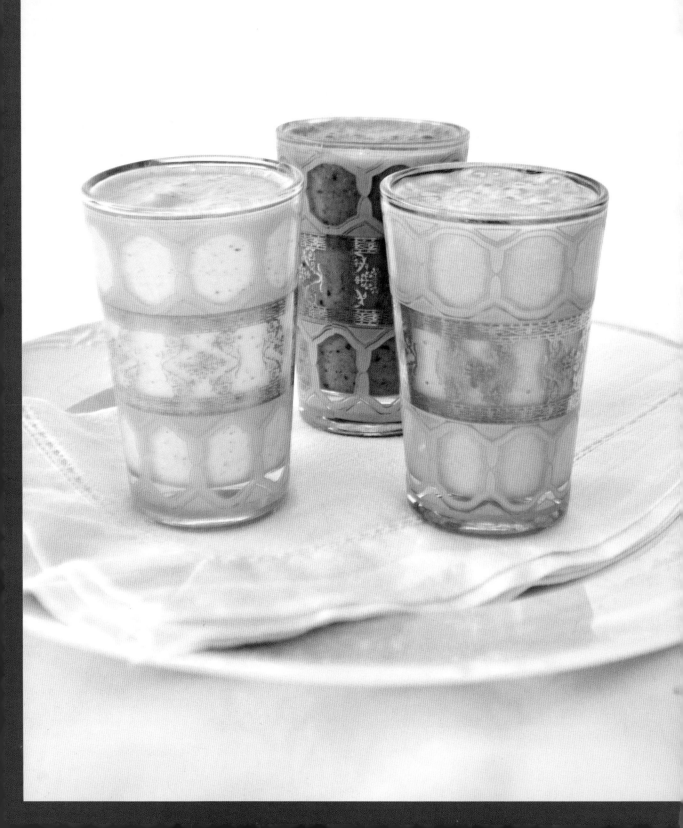

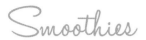
Smoothies

The following five smoothie recipes provide ways to incorporate extra vegetables in your children's diet, while treating them with a refreshing and sweet snack. Try serving in an opaque cup with a lid if fussy with colors of food. All of the recipes serve one child.

Pumpkin, Banana and Honey Smoothie

1 heaped tablespoon
   steamed pumpkin
   (leftovers are ideal)
½ small banana
1 teaspoon honey
pinch ground cinnamon
125 ml (4 fl oz) milk

1. Place all ingredients in a blender and puree until smooth.

Zucchini and Apple Smoothie

⅓ small steamed zucchini
   (courgette) (leftovers are
   ideal)
1 small apple, peeled and
   cored
2 tablespoons Greek style
   yogurt
4 fresh mint leaves

1. Place all ingredients in a blender and puree until smooth.

Beans, Banana and Blueberry Smoothie

5 steamed green beans
   (leftovers are ideal)
½ small banana
1 tablespoon blueberries
   (fresh or frozen)
125 ml (4 fl oz) milk

1. Place all ingredients in a blender and puree until smooth.

Sweet Potato, Prune and Cinnamon Smoothie

2 heaped tablespoons
   steamed sweet potato
   (leftovers are ideal)
3 hydrated pitted prunes
   (cover with water in a
   small ramekin the night
   before to hydrate)
¼ teaspoon ground
   cinnamon
125 ml (4 fl oz) milk

1. Place all ingredients in a blender and puree until smooth.

Carrot and Raspberry Smoothie

1 tablespoon chopped
   steamed carrot (leftovers
   are ideal)
1 heaped tablespoon
   raspberries (fresh or
   frozen)
1 heaped tablespoon Greek
   style yogurt
1 teaspoon honey (optional)

1. Place all ingredients in a blender and puree until smooth.

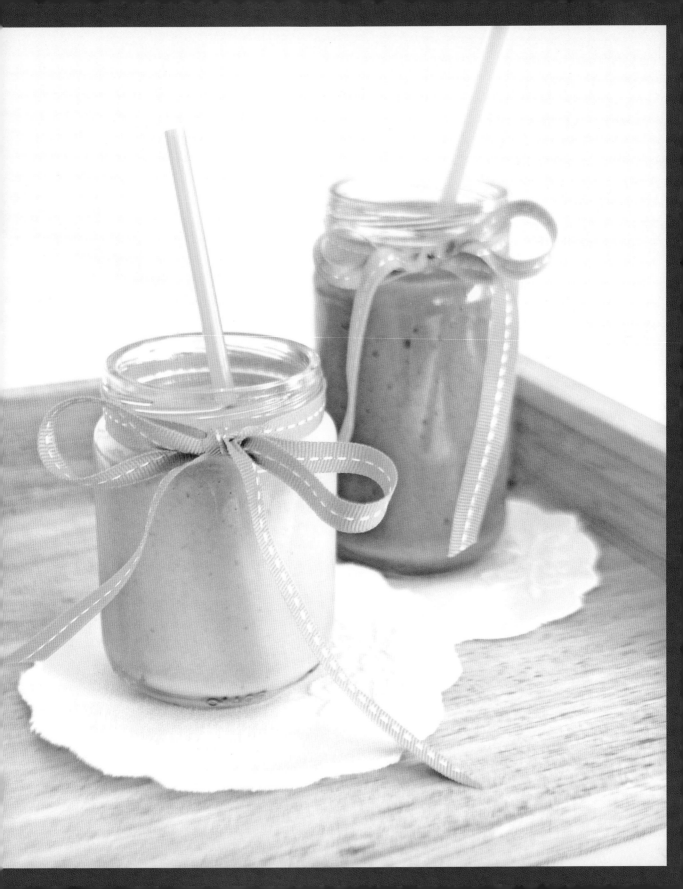

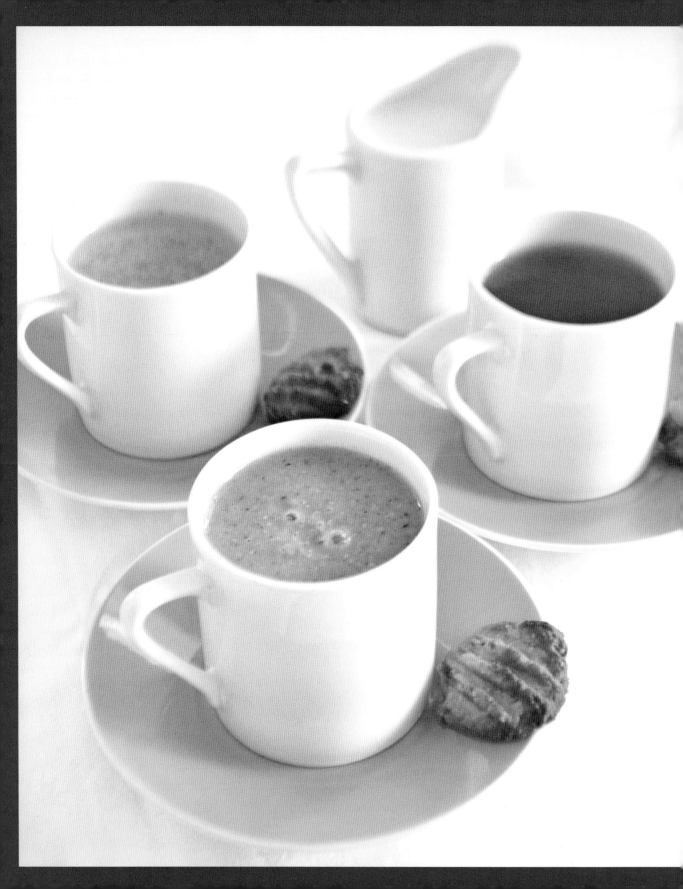

Children's Chai

This is a great drink for young children to have while adults are having cups of tea and coffee. Almond or soy milk can be added for a dairy free alternative.

2 prunes, pitted and cut in thirds
150 ml (5 fl oz) boiling water
1 tablespoon milk
Pinch ground cinnamon

1. Place prunes into a small jug and pour boiling water over the top of them, steep for 15 minutes, stirring occasionally.
2. Using a tea strainer, pour prune tea into a cup, add milk and cinnamon and stir well.

Kiddie Cuppa

This is a tasty morning or afternoon tea drink for the cooler months. Cow's milk can be substituted with soy, almond or rice milk for a dairy free alternative.

1/3 medium banana
2 pitted prunes
1/3 teaspoon cacao or cocoa powder
90 ml (3 fl oz) milk
90 ml (3 fl oz) hot water

1. Place banana, prunes and cacao into a small blender and puree.
2. Add milk and hot water and blend until frothy.
3. Serve in favorite mug or latte cup.

Toddler Toddy

This is a nutritious and soothing warm drink for toddlers or adults. Honey, lemon or ginger can be added for further medicinal purposes.

2 prunes pitted and cut in thirds
150 ml (5 fl oz) boiling water
1 tablespoon fresh orange juice

1. Place prunes into a small jug and pour boiling water over the top of them, steep for 15 minutes, stirring occasionally.
2. Using a tea strainer, pour prune tea into a cup, add orange juice and stir well.

Shakes

These three shakes make one regular or two small sized serves.

Mango and Coconut Shake

1 small mango cheek
1 teaspoon honey
60 ml (2 fl oz) coconut milk
60 ml (2 fl oz) milk

1. Place all ingredients into a blender and blend until smooth and aerated.
2. Pour into one adult glass or two children's glasses.

Berry Bliss Shake

2 teaspoons of mixed
   berries (fresh or frozen)
1 teaspoon honey
150 ml (5 fl oz) milk

1. Place all ingredients into a blender and blend until smooth and aerated.
2. Pour into one adult glass or two children's glasses.

Choc Mint Shake

6 medium sized mint leaves
1 teaspoon cacao or cocoa
   powder
1 teaspoon honey
150 ml (5 fl oz) milk

1. Place mint leaves and 2 tablespoons of milk into a small blender and puree.
2. Add balance of ingredients and blend until frothy.
3. Pour into one adult glass or two children's glasses.

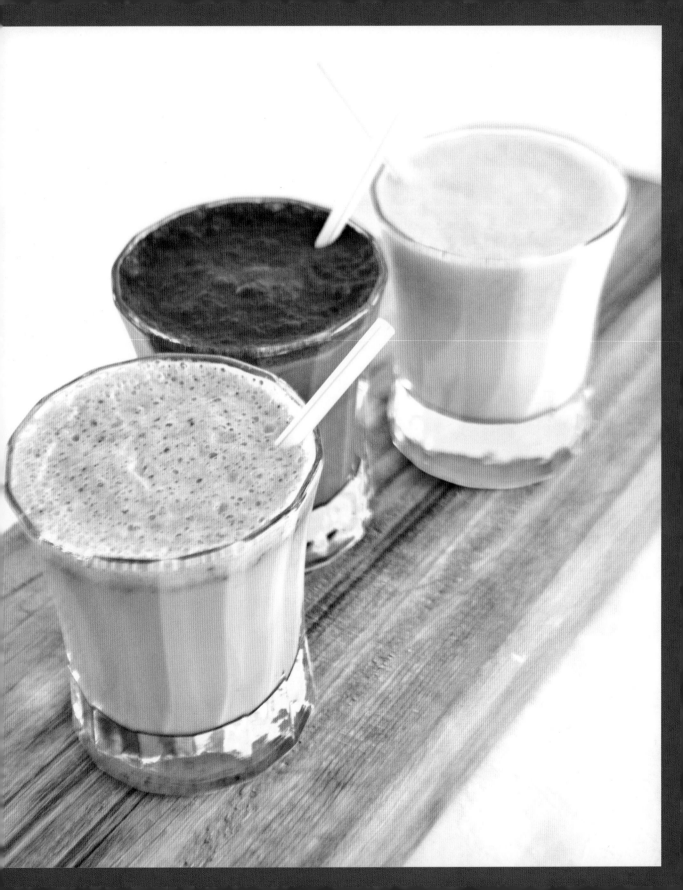

AUTHOR BIOGRAPHY

Cassandra Fenaughty is a qualified health coach, author and founder of *Easy Grub Healthy Bub* – a motivational cooking program for parents.

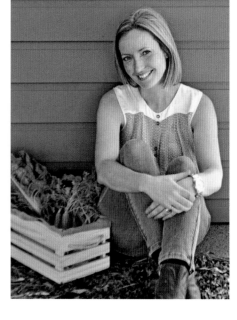

Over twenty years ago Cassandra began working in the bakery industry, later managing a branch of a high-end bakery, catering and confectionery company. When Cassandra and her husband Chris welcomed their first child into the world Cassandra decided to leave her successful career to embark upon the lifelong learning journey of parenthood, in turn returning to her love of food.

Cassandra began recipe writing and researching nutrition as soon as her daughter started eating solids. Being a 'stay at home parent' her recipe designs began to be themed around healthy, simple and affordable cooking to provide her daughter with the best possible start in life.

In 2013 Cassandra established *Easy Grub Healthy Bub*, a simple cookbook and cooking demonstration program for childcare centers showing parents how easy it can be to prepare healthy and affordable food for the family. Cassandra has now completed studies in Nutrition and Diet and provides health coaching and meal planning for families both online and face-to-face. Cassandra's health coaching not only improves family diets and well-being but helps families lower their grocery bills.

Numerous Community Centers, Community Organizations and Marketplaces now commission Cassandra to not only teach parents and caregivers how to cook, but to explain why good nutrition is so important for children, how much money can be saved by home cooking, and how to cook efficiently with programs such as 'Two weeks of Snacks in 90 minutes' and 'Easy Dinners'.

Through working with various community groups, Cassandra's passion for helping families to become healthier is fuelled by hearing endless stories of food related behavioral problems, parents who have never been taught to cook and only know packaged and processed foods and busy working parents who want the best for their children and can't find the time.

ACKNOWLEDGEMENTS

This book wouldn't have been possible without help from my wonderful husband who looked after our daughter while I cooked another dish and raced around taking photos of it! I also want to thank my Mother for helping babysit, cook and listen to my ideas as this book unfolded. Of course my biggest thank you goes to my beautiful daughter for taste testing all the food and inspiring me to provide other mothers with the opportunity to give their children the best start in life. Lastly I'd like to thank all my family and friends who helped me cook, trial recipes, proofread, brainstorm, lend props for photos and babysit – there are too many to mention, but you all know who you are!

Author Photography: Leah Hermann

REFERENCES

Beck, K 2015, *Certificate of Nutrition and Diet, Beck Health and Nutrition*, Collaroy Beach, Australia.

National Health and Medical Research Council, 2003, *Dietary Guidelines for Children and Adolescents in Australia*, AGPS, Canberra, Australia.

Index

T

V

W

First published in 2016 by New Holland Publishers Pty Ltd
London • Sydney • Auckland

The Chandlery Unit 704 50 Westminster Bridge Road London SE1 7QY United Kingdom
1/66 Gibbes Street Chatswood NSW 2067 Australia
5/39 Woodside Ave Northcote, Auckland 0627 New Zealand

www.newhollandpublishers.com

A record of this book is held at the British Library and the National Library of Australia.

ISBN 9781742578439

Managing Director: Fiona Schultz
Publisher: Diane Ward
Project Editor: Anna Brett
Designer: Lorena Susak
Typesetter: Peter Guo
Production Director: Olga Dementiev
Printer: Toppan Leefung Printing Limited

10 9 8 7 6 5 4 3 2 1

Keep up with New Holland Publishers on Facebook
www.facebook.com/NewHollandPublishers

US: $24.99
UK: £14.99